T0272760

TIMING IN THE FIGHTING ARTS

Your guide to winning in the ring and surviving on the street

TIMING IN THE FIGHTING ARTS
Your guide to winning in the ring and surviving on the street

Loren W. Christensen

Wim Demeere

YMAA Publication Center, Inc.
Wolfeboro, NH USA

YMAA Publication Center, Inc.
PO Box 480
Wolfeboro, NH 03894
800 669-8892 • www.ymaa.com • info@ymaa.com

Paperback ISBN: 9781594394966 (print) • ISBN: 9781594394973 (ebook)

All rights reserved including the right of reproduction in whole or in part in any form.
Copyright © 2004, 2016 by Loren W. Christensen and Wim Demeere

20200325

Publisher's Cataloging in Publication

Christensen, Loren W.
 Timing in the fighting arts : your guide to winning in the ring and surviving on the street / by
Loren W. Christensen, Wim Demeere.--
1st ed.
   p. cm.
 ISBN 9781594394966
 1. MArtial arts--Training. 2. Speed. I. Demeere, Wim. II. Title.
 GV1102.7.T7C46 2004
 796.8--dc22

                          2016944170

The author and publisher of the material are NOT RESPONSIBLE in any manner whatsoever
for any injury that may occur through reading or following the instructions in this manual.

The activities, physical or otherwise, described in this manual may be too strenuous or dangerous for some people, and the reader(s) should consult a physician before engaging in them.

Warning: While self-defense is legal, fighting is illegal. If you don't know the difference,
you'll go to jail because you aren't defending yourself. You are fighting—or worse. Readers
are encouraged to be aware of all appropriate local and national laws relating to self-defense,
reasonable force, and the use of weaponry, and act in accordance with all applicable laws at all
times. Understand that while legal definitions and interpretations are generally uniform, there
are small—but very important—differences from state to state and even city to city. To stay out
of jail, you need to know these differences. Neither the author nor the publisher assumes any
responsibility for the use or misuse of information contained in this book.

Nothing in this document constitutes a legal opinion, nor should any of its contents be treated
as such. While the author believes everything herein is accurate, any questions regarding
specific self-defense situations, legal liability, and/or interpretation of federal, state, or local laws
should always be addressed by an attorney at law.

When it comes to martial arts, self-defense, and related topics, no text, no matter how well
written, can substitute for professional, hands-on instruction. **These materials should be used
for academic study only.**

Printed in USA

Contents

Introduction   9

Chapter One: The Nuts and Bolts of Timing   18

Physical components   19
The OODA loop   26
You and OODA   29
Types of reactions   37
Hick's Law 46
Mental components 53
Seizing an opportunity   61
It's called timing for a reason   77

Chapter Two: Winning & Surviving Takes Perfect Timing

Fighting ranges   82
Don't "overpull" your blows 92
Positioning 98
Framing with footwork   102
Centerline   104
Your fighting posture   112
Slow? Improve your timing   126
Timing when you are already fast   134
Age, injuires and speed   140
How to use timing to increase your power   149
Know the power of your weapons   152
Eliminate excess movements 155
The value of experience and how to get it   157
What to do when you can't use footwork   162

Chapter Three: Into the Mean Streets   174

Two techniques that almost always save your bacon   175
Verbal Judo 177
Know when it's time to get physical 181
Timing against big guys   197
Timing against a gun threat   209
Timing against the blade   212
Fighting multiple opponents   214

Chapter Four: It works in a tournament, but will it work in the street? 226

"That would never happen on the street"   228
Sport techniques for the street   232
Punching the body   238
High kicks in the street   242

Chapter Five: Timing a grab: How to close the gap   246

Law enforcement needs this, too   247
The setting   247
1. Move when he is distracted   248
2. When he changes stances   249
3. Catch him with his feet parallel   250
4. When he drops his hands   251
5. When moving back   252
6. When he retracts his attack   253
7. When he is talking   254
8. When you are with a buddy   255
Doing your civic duty   257

Chapter Six: Wisdom of the ages   258

The Tai Chi Chuan Classics   260
The Art of War   264
A Book of Five Rings   268

Chapter Seven: Drills   274

Dodge the stick   274
Ball dodging   276
Back to the wall   277
Touch and go   278
Surprise attack   279
Stop the bag   280
The fan drill   281
Pin the glove to the wall   283
Yardstick   284
React to the string   285
Hand mitts hitting drill   286
Rhythm kicking drill   287
Timing a feint   287

Baiting   288
Catch the rabbit   289

Conclusion   **290**

Dedication

Loren W. Christensen: To my incredible children, Carrie, Dan, Amy, and my granddaughter, Dakota. Know that good timing will get you far in life.

Wim Demeere: To my children, Lauren and Xander, who I love more than words can express.

Acknowledgements

Many thanks to our patient models

Amy Christensen	Mark Whited
Jace Widmer	Tim Sukimoto
Lisa Place	Gary Sussman
Rock Dehon	Dirk Crokaert
Jaques	

The two really, really good looking models are Loren and Wim

Our photographers

Amy Christensen	Gary Sussman
Lisa Place	Lana McKay
Fiorella Notarianni	Gerd Morren
Lotfi El Garim	Andy Benfield

Authors and teachers who contributed to this book

Alain Burrese, author of *Hard-Won Wisdom From The School of Hard Knocks*; *Hapkido Hoshinsul* (video), and *Streetfighting Essentials* (video)
Website: www.burrese.com

Prof. Dan Anderson, 7th Dan American Freestyle Karate, 6th Dan Modern Arnis, 4-time National Top Ten Champion Fighter, 2002 Funakoshi Shotokan Karate World Champion. Author of: *American Freestyle Karate: A Guide to Sparring, Tactics and Strategies (American Freestyle Karate vol. 2*; and *Advanced Modern Arnis: A Road to Mastery* Website: www.danandersonkarate

Bob Orlando, author of *Martial Art America: A Western approach to Eastern Arts, Indonesian Fighting Fundamentals; Fighting Arts of Indonesia* (video); *Reflex Action: Training Drills to Fighting Skills* (video); and *Fighting Footwork of Kuntao and Silat* (video) Website: www.orlandokuntao.com

Frank Garza, 3rd Degree Black Belt American Kenpo Karate

Larry Kwolek, 2nd Dan Aikido, 1st Dan Aiki toho Iai. Website: www. Aikidojo.info

Marc "Animal" MacYoung, author of *Cheap Shots, Ambushes, and Other Lessons: A Down-and-Dirty Book on Streetfighting and Survival; Fists, Wits, and a Wicked Right: Surviving on the Wild Side of the Street; Knives, Knife Fighting, and Related Hassles: How to Survive a Real Knife Fight; Pool Cues, Beer Bottles, and Baseball Bats: Animal's Guide to Improvised Weapons for Self-Defense and Survival;* and *Winning a Street Knife Fight: Realistic Offensive Techniques.*

Mark Hatmaker, expert in Western martial arts (boxing/pugilism/all-in submission wrestling) and sport specific combat conditioning, and author of *No Holds Barred Fighting: The Ultimate Guide to Submission Wrestling* as well as numerous instructional videos including: The *ESP Raw Series, The Gladiator Conditioning Program; Extreme Boxing; The ABC'S OF NHB; Beyond Brazilian Jiu-Jitsu* and many more. For more information about Mark Hatmaker and Western Martial Arts see his webpage at www. extremeselfprotection.com

Martina Sprague, author of *Fighting Science and The Science of Takedowns, Throws & Grappling for Self-defense* Website: www.modernfighter.com

Michael Janich, author of *Fighting Folders: The Definitive Guide to Personal Defense with Tactical Folding Knives; Advanced Fighting Folders: State-of-the-Art Training and Tactics for the Defensive Use of Tactical Folding Knives; Blowguns: The Breath of Death; Breath of Death: The Blowgun Video* and *Street Steel: Choosing and Carrying Self-Defense Knives.* **Website: www. martialbladecraft.net**

Stefan Stennud, 6th Dan Aikido, 4th Dan Iaido Website: http://www. stenudd.com

"A GOOD PLAN VIOLENTLY EXECUTED RIGHT NOW
IS FAR BETTER THAN A PERFECT PLAN EXECUTED NEXT WEEK."

~ GENERAL GEORGE S. PATTON

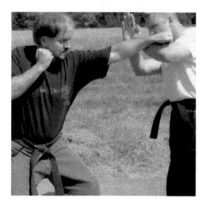

INTRODUCTION

Although timing, precise timing, is the most critical of all martial arts fighting components, it's often pushed in the background in favor of stretching, bag work, forms, and reps before a mirror. While flexibility from stretching, power from bag work, precision movement from forms, and speed and coordination from rep practice are certainly important, they are of little value if you can't get your technique to the target at the right moment. With an understanding of timing - knowing when to hit, where to hit, and with which weapon to hit - you dramatically increase your ability to use those well-trained kicks, punches and blocks, and defeat even those fighters possessing speed and power superior to yours. Imagine their amazement. Imagine yours!

If you happen to be exceptionally fast and strong, your timing will be even better when you have a greater understanding of all its facets. Why? Because good speed allows you to take advantage of even the briefest moment of opportunity, and good strength allows you to affect more damage when your blow hits the target.

Then comes Father Time. As it passes, and you get older, your speed and strength begin to wane. What do you do then? First, don't fret about it. Second, reach into the bag of timing tricks crammed into this book and you are good to go long into your retirement years.

What is precise timing?

Seems like a simple enough question, but the answer is big, real big. In fact, this entire book is the answer. For now, let's say that timing is the skill and art of choosing the precise moment to hit, grab, back off, or say the right thing to bring the threat of a fight, or a fight in progress, to a conclusion in your favor. Timing is the ability to take advantage of *a window of opportunity*. While that phrase is a cliché, one that you are going to see over and over throughout this book, it fits our subject matter perfectly. Whether your opponent inadvertently opens a window for you, or you cleverly create a moment that forces him to open it, that is the instant you attack. That is timing.

Here are three real-life situations in which timing was absolutely critical.

*

When co-author Christensen was a police officer, he once faced a mountain of a man on the center span of one of the many high bridges that cross the mighty Willamette River in Portland, Oregon. Five minutes earlier, the radio call reported that a six-feet six, 250-pound man had gone berserk inside a tavern and hurt several patrons before he had fled in the direction of the bridge. Although four officers had been dispatched, Christensen got to the bridge first and spotted the big man lumbering along. He pulled his patrol car to the curb a few feet in front of the giant and asked dispatch to have his backup officers hurry.

"Hold it right there," Christensen ordered, after he had exited his car and stepped up on the sidewalk.

The man ignored the command and advanced with a gait not unlike Boris Karloff's in the original *Frankenstein* movie.

Christensen and the giant stood on the sidewalk at the apex of the bridge, with six busy traffic lanes on one side of them, and on the other, a four-foot railing, then a 60-foot drop into the raging Willamette River.

The giant's facial expression read, "You're gonna take a swim, cop," and he stopped for a moment, as if to underscore his threatening look.

Christensen thought of the 30 pounds of gear he was wearing: No, swimming was not an option today. He needed a different plan, but considering the guy's size, what would it be?

The big guy lumbered forward again, and Christensen stepped back once, twice, three times. When a blaring horn distracted the giant for half a second, Christensen seized the moment and slid his baton from its belt ring, holding it out of sight behind his rear leg. "Stop!" Christensen commanded, but the man kept coming, raising his arms forward, reaching, just like the stalking Frankenstein monster. Christensen knew he was going to have to fight him, but he also knew it was a good idea to "soften" him first.

Just as the man's extended hands got within range, his eyes darted to the side at a passing, noisy truck. Another moment. Another window of opportunity, opening just a crack and ever so briefly. Christensen whipped his baton in a blurry arc into the thick, stubby fingers of the giant's closest hand.

The big guy belched a curse and snapped his wounded hand back against his chest, covering it with his other and bending forward at the waist in pain. In one motion, Christensen stabbed his baton back into its ring holder, grabbed the man's huge head and yanked him forcefully onto his belly. Backup officers screeched to the curb and, a moment later, they had wrestled the man into handcuffs.

That is perfect timing.

*

Once in a full-contact competition, Demeere noticed that his first opponent of the day held his hands low even when moving into range. So, Demeere began kicking the man's legs and punching his body to keep his attention low so he could score a big hit up high. The plan worked. The next time his opponent moved into range with his hands down to guard against the low blows, Demeere seized the moment to use a fast, hard spinning hook kick to snap the man's head back and make him see little chirping birds swirl about his dazed skull. The man recovered a few minutes later but was too shaken to continue.

Demeere's next opponent was much taller than him, and he too didn't protect his head well, probably thinking that he didn't need to because of the reach difference. So Demeere simply used the same tactic as before: attack low to keep the man's mind and hands down and then hit him high for the score. The next time his opponent made the mistake of stepping in with a low guard, Demeere waited until the range was just right and then executed a fake-double-jump front kick that just nicked his opponent in the eye socket, but hard enough to TKO the man and win the match.

That is perfect timing.

*

It's unknown why the deranged man walked into the trailer park that day and it's unknown why he smashed his way into the middle-aged woman's trailer. It is known that he was armed with a shotgun and that his mental turmoil had pushed him into a killing rage. He greeted the frightened woman with his fist, smashing her nose to one side, sending her sprawling. Although she could not have fathomed the violation that would happen to her, within five minutes her world was to turn so horrific and so despicable that even jaded, veteran cops would be stunned.

The madman ripped her clothes away and then, in an act of total depravity, inserted the barrel of the shotgun into her body and duct taped it into place. Ignoring her piercing screams, he then duct taped his hand to the weapon and his finger into the trigger. And for the next two hours, he ranted, most of it gibberish, all of it fiery, hate-filled and deadly.

Outside, the police were in place. A hostage negotiator talked on the phone with the suspect and a police sniper had taken a position where he could see the front window. Every few seconds, the man, his arm around the woman's neck, would pass by the window.

His rage began to boil over, his screams turned unintelligible except for his threats to pull the trigger -- those were chillingly clear. Outside, several yards away and behind cover, a police sniper watched the trailer's little window through his riflescope. His orders: Take the shot at the first clear opportunity.

The sniper knew that not only did the opportunity have to be precise and sufficient, but the bullet had to hit what police call an "idealized target," one that would end the man's life so fast that it would prevent a reflexive motor action, meaning that he would die instantly. Doctors say that such a precise hit causes "flaccid paralysis," in that all of the recipient's muscles suddenly relax so that he is incapable of any motion thereafter, such as a reflexive pull of the trigger.

For 20 minutes the sniper watched the man and woman pass by the window, but never was there the right target at the right moment. Then the suspect passed by the window once more, and for just a hairbreadth of a second, he turned his head just right – exposing the idealized target.

The high-caliber round ripped through the man's brain stem, terminating his life force instantaneously – so that his trigger finger died at the same moment he did.

And the woman lived.

That is perfect timing.

In Christensen's situation on the bridge, there were several moments involving timing. Christensen says that it was bad timing that he found the suspect without the benefit of his backup being on the scene. It was good timing that allowed him to draw his baton unseen, and it was good timing that allowed him to strike the suspect when he was momentarily distracted. In Demeere's full-contact fights, he took advantage of his opponents' errors by ensuring that they continued to err. Then when time and distance were perfect, when the window of opportunity opened, Demeere sent them to Sleepville City. In the hostage incident, the police sniper had the harrowing responsibility to terminate a potential killer's life without the suspect inadvertently and reflexively ending the hostage's life. Timing was based on one tiny fraction of a second when a precise target came into view.

Your authors have been there and done that. Wim Demeere began training in the martial arts as a teenager and over the years studied a variety of fighting systems that have helped him come out on top in the mean streets and bring home the gold in grueling full-contact fighting events in his native country of Belgium and throughout the world. As a personal trainer, he teaches, trains and advises clients on health, exercise and the fighting arts.

Loren W. Christensen began training in karate and jujitsu in 1965 at the age of 19. Since then he has used his skills to win over 50 tournaments and to survive deadly confrontations as a military policeman in Saigon, Vietnam and as a police officer for 25 years in Portland, Oregon. He has written and taught extensively on post-traumatic stress disorder, the psychology and physiology of combat, martial arts training, and police work.

Together, Wim Demeere and Loren Christensen co-authored the best selling book *The Fighter's Body: An Owner's Manual.*

Here are just a few of the goodies you are going to learn about timing.

- What functions occur in your brain when a timing moment happens? Learn about them here and how to make them work faster for you.

- How important is speed for successful timing? Learn why many experts say you don't have to be fast at all.

- What the heck is the OODA loop? Learn how understanding it dramatically increases your timing ability and makes your opponent's life miserable.

- What are natural blocks? Learn why they are faster and increase your timing speed.

- What is Hick's Law? Learn how violating it can get you hurt.

- What are circles of influence? Learn how understanding them helps you hit at just the right moment.

- Can you control your opponent's spine? Learn how doing it provides you with more time to attack.

- Can precise timing make your blows more powerful? Yes. Learn how easy it is to do.

- Can you apply defensive timing while seated in your car? Yes. Learn how hundreds of pounds of steel can be used to stop an attacker.

- Do you know what objects can be used as weapons no matter where you are? Learn where and what they are and, most importantly, *when* to use them.

- What are the timing considerations against a knife or gun? What you learn here just might save your life.

- Will tournament point-fighting techniques work against a street assailant? Learn why the authors say yes, but with an explanation.

- What must you know about timing to survive against multiple opponents? Learn when to strike each opponent.

- What are the timing tricks law enforcement officers use? Discover how they can work for you.

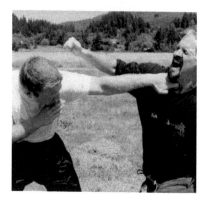

CHAPTER ONE

THE NUTS AND BOLTS OF TIMING

Him slow, you fast: a winning combination

In the Introduction, we said that one definition of timing is the act of taking advantage of a *window of opportunity,* a term used frequently in the pages that follow. In this chapter, we discuss the basic components that exist in a timing moment and all that goes into taking advantage of that moment. Understanding the core elements of timing in this chapter helps you better use the information in subsequent pages.

If you have read our book *The Fighter's Body: An Owner's Manual,* you know that we don't get caught up in mysticism and gobblygook, elements often used and abused in martial arts literature. We won't do it here, either. Actually, there really isn't anything mystical about timing, although when done right it can appear to be so. Timing is just a matter of understanding how various components interact with each other and with other aspects of fighting.

It's been our experience as trainers that many fighters perceive timing as just "something you do," like tying on their belts and saluting to their partners. However, by not understanding the significance and totality of timing, they fail to reach their full potential because they inadvertently neglect certain components, or they don't use them simply because they don't even know they exist. What follows is an overview of what goes on "behind the scenes" when you time your front kick just right and it slams into the gut of an onrushing opponent like a kick from an elephant (if elephants do indeed kick). Keep this thought in mind: *Theory without practice is useless as is practice without theory.* So let's start with the theory before getting all bone-crushingly practical.

Physical components

In the context of martial arts, timing is influenced by the way your body is hardwired to react to stimuli. Your ol' bod' has several systems in place to take care of this, systems that are linked to each other. Consider your senses, in particular your sight, touch and hearing.

- You *see* an opponent shift his weight for a kick and you react by exploding into him with a punch.

- You *feel* your opponent pulling at you during a clinch, and you yield to the pull adding a technique of your own.

- You *hear* running footsteps behind you and you spin around, your guard up and ready.

In each of these examples, one of your senses perceived the information and sent that data on a neurological pathway to your brain where it was perceived as critical. A split-second decision was made to react in a given manner, which resulted in your successful response. In each of the three examples (and any others you can think of), the first of several steps in the process of perceiving and reacting begins with your senses.

Nervous systems

Once the information has been gathered by one of your senses, the data is fired to the brain via the peripheral and central nervous systems -- which are basically networks connected to everything in your body -- where the info is processed. These networks allow the brain to receive information, decipher it, decide what to do, and then issue out commands to your muscles.

The brain

Although it's beyond the scope of this book to detail the function of each specific part of the brain, it's important that you have at least a rudimentary understanding of how your gray matter functions when it comes to seizing a timing moment. Later, when we give you drills and exercises to improve your ability to hit at the right time, you will have a better idea how your brain functions in relation to the physical process that makes for optimum timing. Here it is in the proverbial nutshell.

A very busy place, your brain Once information has been observed or otherwise perceived – say, you see a big haymaker punch arcing toward your snout – the data is sent laser-quick to your brain via your nervous system, where it's quickly analyzed so a decision can be made as to how to respond. Depending on a number of factors, analyzing takes place in several areas of the brain.

A crucial element for you to know is that under the stress of a real-life street altercation, other parts of your brain -- parts other than those involved in a regular training session – jump into action and play an important role in your survival. Research suggests that higher brain functions, such as those that occur in your conscious mind, are sometimes bypassed when you are suddenly confronted with real danger. Instead, the information is relayed directly to a primitive part of your brain called the amygdala, one you inherited from your prehistoric ancestors. It has only one thing on it's, uh, mind: your survival. In other words, it wants desperately to keep your bacon out of the fire. It isn't capable of complicated decisions, but those it does make are reached more quickly than those made by your conscious mind. When microseconds can mean the difference between life and death, a high-speed system makes a lot of sense. Now, this doesn't mean that higher brain functions aren't used when fighting, but it does mean that under extreme stress it's probable that you will react differently than you do in class. More on this later.

Here is what happens after the analysis is completed. The brain has recognized the attack as not a good thing and picks a response. It might choose for you to evade the attack, execute a block, freeze and scream like a little child, or any one of several other possibilities. You react in whatever fashion because your brain has sent a set of instructions back down your nervous system to whichever set of muscles are to be used, or to your vocal cords if you are a screamer.

Are you training correctly?

All the steps that occur in the brain are crucial to choosing and executing a correct response to a given attack. Yet a large number of martial artists spend the majority of their time working on the last step, physical execution. They repeat endless repetitions of punches, kicks and blocks in an effort to become fast and powerful. Though such training is important, they are missing a phase that helps them better use these highly developed weapons. They need to develop the various steps that occur in the brain *that precede* their kicks, blocks and punches. Not until all phases have been developed will they possess impeccable timing.

Don't fret, because that is what this book is all about.

Muscles and movement speed

If all functions in your nervous system are normal and your brain functions well, your perception, analysis and decision making can be developed to an extraordinary level of speed. With the right training, you can pick the correct response to an attack in less time than it takes to blink your eyes. Then you must execute your technique fast enough to get to the target before the opportunity goes away, and land with enough power to cause grief. This is where your bulging, tattooed muscles come into play. They are the last stage and the deciding factor as to how fast you execute your punches, kicks, blocks and evasions.

The type of muscle fibers you have plays an important role here. There are several kinds. The most interesting ones for our purposes are called fast-twitch muscle fibers, aptly named because they contract explosively and enable your muscles to generate tremendous strength and speed. The bad news is that there is little you can do about the quantity of fast-twitch muscle fibers you have in relation to the other types. The little suckers are genetically determined, so blame your parents if they didn't give you many. Lucky kids are born with large percentages of fast-twitch muscle fiber and tend to excel at sports where speed is essential, such as sprinting and the martial arts. Those born with more slow-twitch muscle fibers are better suited for long distance running, or activities that require great endurance but less raw power and speed.

The good news is that though you might be cursed with a low percentage of fast-twitch muscles, you can still be quick and have great timing. The bad news is that you have to work hard to reach that level because your technical skills have to be better than those fighters with predominantly fast-twitch muscles. In particular, you must work to eliminate all excess movement. Excess, for our purposes here, is defined as movement that isn't necessary for the delivery of your techniques. Get rid of the baggage and you might be faster than you think, maybe even faster than your opponent.

Kuntao-Silat expert Bob Orlando said this about fast-twitch muscles: "I am not naturally fast because I don't have fast twitch muscle fibers. However, I am "quick" because I work hard on the two main components of speed: Relaxation and good lines." Co-author Demeere once hosted a seminar with Mr. Orlando and can attest to his quickness. He is neither too tense nor too relaxed. He knows how to contract his muscles precisely for optimal speed. At the same time, he has no noticeable excess movement in his techniques, something he calls "good lines." Demeere was nearly 30 years younger than Orlando, but he found himself unable to match Orlando's speed and technical accuracy.

Reacting to a stimulus

Let's examine more closely the components involved when you react to a stimulus; think of it as a chain of events that occurs every time you launch a technique. Understanding them will help you later when examining the many drills in this book, especially those seemingly strange ones that work individual parts of the chain. By working these drills, you improve each component that makes up the whole chain. Understand that if you choose to work only on one drill for one component, the others will be a weak link in your response time. We talk more about this later, but for now know that you need to train them all to gain optimum reaction time in competition or in the street. As the saying goes: The chain is only as strong as its weakest link. Here is the entire chain:

- The receptor -- eye, ear or touch -- receives a stimulus: You *see* a punch; you *hear* footsteps behind you; you *feel* a hand grab your shoulder from behind.

- That information is transmitted to the brain.

- The brain analyzes the stimulus.

- A response is formulated (the fewer choices, the faster the response. This is discussed in detail later).

- The selected response is transferred via the nervous system to the muscles.

- The muscles contract and the response is executed (block, punch or run).

Increase speed by eliminating wasted movement

A beginner often cocks or chambers his arm prior to punching, usually by lifting his fist and drawing it back before launching it at the target. When fractions of seconds are critical to the outcome of a fight, such actions are a waste of time and alert the opponent to what is coming. It's far better to simply explode that fist forward without any preparation at all.

Launching an attack without excess movement, without telegraphing, is often referred to as "looking sharp" or "having clean technique." If your opponent, who is gifted with fast-twitch muscle fibers, wastes time by adding useless movements to his techniques, you can beat him to the punch with sharp, efficient techniques, though technically you might be slower.

Response time

The more quickly you respond, the greater the chance you will be the victor. Response time is divided into two more segments: (1) Reaction time, which determines how fast you react to a stimulus; (2) movement time, which is the time it takes from the beginning of the movement to its conclusion.

Reaction time This is the time needed for the brain to register the stimulus and decide on a response. Your brain has to process the information it receives and then determine what to do with the data. For our purposes it can be subdivided into three more categories.

- **Sensation:** The amount of time it takes to register a stimulus. Several factors influence this: The higher the intensity of the stimulus (louder, bigger, bold) the faster your reaction time. For example, you react more quickly to a visual directly in front of you than you do to one in your periphery. It's believed that auditory cues are perceived faster than visual ones.

- **Perception:** In the previous stage, you perceived a sudden movement. In this one you must identify exactly what that movement is. Say it's a punch rocketing toward your face. Your brain quickly searches its memory banks to compare this information against everything else it knows to determine if a punch is a good thing or a bad thing. If the punch catches you by surprise because you didn't see its initial launch (you don't see it until it's two inches from your face), or it's a technique you have never faced before, you will probably react more slowly. Though it's possible that you will instinctively try to move away from the danger before you fully realize what it is, your counter technique will still be slower than if you had seen the technique in plain sight and recognized it clearly.

- **Response selection and programming:** This last stage concerns the amount of time it takes to pick a response and to program its movement. The more signals you are presented, the harder it becomes to react quickly. For example, if a fighter attacks you like an octopus with what seems like five arms and six legs all coming in a flurry, your response will be slower than if the attack were a single, looping punch. However, if you know there are only one or two possible attacks coming, your response will be much faster. For example, if your opponent's back is to a wall, you know he can only come straight at you or move to the left or right.

Practice plays a significant role, too. In essence, the more you practice a response, the more you improve its neural pathways, and the faster it will be.

Movement time

The information has been analyzed and processed, a course of action has been decided upon, and all systems are ready for your muscles to execute the plan. How fast you move is influenced by a number of factors, such as these:

- **Adrenaline** When experiencing the emotional and adrenal stress of a high-risk situation, gross motor skills are performed faster than fine-motor skills. In extreme cases, generally when your stress-induced heart rate reaches 145 beats a minute and higher, fine motor skills are impossible to perform. A downward hammer fist is a gross motor skill technique. Most intricate, fancy-smancy techniques are defined as fine-motor skills.

- **Arousal** This refers to your state of readiness, that is, the amount of muscular tension you have throughout your body. In subsequent paragraphs, we cover the mental aspects of arousal and how quality training can keep yours at a minimum. Experiments have determined that an intermediate level of arousal yields the best reaction times. If you are too tight or too loose, reaction times begin to increase. Obviously, the "right" level of arousal will differ from person to person.

- **Keep it simple** Though hard and diligent practice increases your speed, know that the more complex the response, the slower it will be, especially when your adrenaline is boiling and your arousal level is into the red zone. *Simple movements are performed more quickly.*

Studies concerning how we react to stimuli have been conducted for years, and though there is still a lot to discover, there is a large amount of information available now. Here are several pieces of info that are directly related to your ability to respond in a fight:

- **Expectation** If you expect a specific stimulus - you know your opponent is going to throw a right backfist - your reaction will be faster than if you are surprised by the attack or faced with an unknown type of attack.

- **Cognitive load** This is a fancy term meaning that the more you divide your attention, the harder it is to react swiftly. If you are reciting a poem, balancing a dinner plate on your toes, and juggling two beach balls in one hand, it will be hard for your brain to see an incoming punch. You have only so much processing power. Often muggers and street fighters unconsciously use this strategy against you by trying to distract or diminish your mental processing power before they launch their attack. For example, they might first ask you directions and when you hesitate to think about it, they attack.

- **The influence of age** Presently, the data isn't entirely conclusive, but what exists suggests that we do get a little slower with age (for this they needed a study?). However, there is the compensating factor of experience that can overcome any decrease in reaction time and movement speed. Martial arts and fitness author Mark Hatmaker says, "It is probably more likely for older martial artists to experience good timing as timing is encultured by long years of inculcation. The more time one puts into efficient training the better the timing is going to be." Martial arts author Martina Sprague agrees: "Older martial artists can have good timing, not only because they may be more experienced than their younger counterparts, but also because older people are not necessarily slow, unresponsive, etc., and timing involves more than speed. Timing involves your ability to be precise with the speed that you do have."

- **Nature of the stimulus** When you defend against an attack, your brain, among other functions, must calculate its trajectory and then plot a defensive maneuver. Though this sounds easy, it can be quite difficult because not all motion is easy to see. Your eyes have a much harder time tracking movement that comes straight towards your face than it does seeing something that cuts across your field of vision. This means that a straight punch is harder to track than a circular one. Similarly, if the attack comes from an angle that is hard to detect, it will likely hit you before you can defend against it. For example, say that as you look at your opponent's face he launches a fast punch from below your field of vision. By the time you see and identify the movement, his fist is likely to have acquired a speed advantage over your reaction time. In other words, you are going to be spitting out teeth.

- **Fatigue** Mental fatigue and sleepiness increases response time, especially with complex tasks, such as blocking multiple attackers or defending against fast combinations from one opponent. Studies show that the effects of 24 hours without sleep on your body and mind is the equivalent of being legally drunk. It's important that we all get sufficient sleep, even more for people working in high-risk occupations, such as police officers, bodyguards, bouncers and soldiers.

- **Warning indicators**   When you know by certain indicators that an attack is imminent, it's easier to react than if you get no warning at all. The indicator might be overt or it might be something you deduce yourself. An example of an overt indicator would be when a drunken brawler shouts, "I'm gonna knock your block off!" as he steps toward you. You think, *Thanks for the tip, dummy, I'm so ready for you.* An example of one that you deduce would be when you notice a potential attacker subtly shifting his weight back, an indicator that provides you with an extra fraction of a second to plan to jam his kick or prepare to block and counter. We talk more about this later.

The OODA loop

Don't let the odd acronym OODA cause you to skip over this section. We refer back to it from time to time throughout this book so it's important that you understand it.

Sometimes called "Boyd's cycle," the OODA loop provides a practical framework to help you use the just-discussed physical aspects of timing. As a martial artist, understanding the OODA loop, and using it to your advantage and to the disadvantage of your opponent, helps you improve your effectiveness in a street encounter, tournament, and in school sparring, and then helps you better evaluate your actions afterwards.

Who was Boyd and what is OODA?

The late Colonel John Boyd, a United States Air Force Korean combat veteran and military tactics scholar, discovered several similarities in wars and in individual battles. His most striking discovery was that when Side A presented Side B with an unexpected and threatening situation, it allowed Side A time and opportunity to gain an advantage. If Side B couldn't adapt to the new situation, B would eventually be defeated since decisions and actions that are delayed are often rendered ineffective due to the constantly changing circumstances of a fight. This led Boyd to the conclusion that conflict is in essence a time-based problem. Whichever side is capable of being quicker at completing the OODA -- Observation-Orientation-Decision-Action -- loop is the one most likely to come out victorious. This cycle can be found in all manners of violent confrontations, whether it's all-out war or simple hand-to-hand combat.

Captain Sid Heal of the Los Angeles Sheriff's Department, scholar, author and researcher, introduces Boyd's work this way: "According to Boyd's theory, conflict can be seen as a series of time-competitive, Observation-Orientation-Decision-Action (OODA) cycles. Each party in a conflict begins by observing themselves, their adversary, and their physical surroundings. Next they orient themselves. Orientation refers to making a mental image or snapshot of the situation. Orientation is necessary because the fluid and chaotic nature of conflicts makes it impossible to process information as fast as we can observe it. This requires a freeze-frame concept and provides a perspective or orientation. Once we have an orientation, we need to make a decision. The decision takes into account all the factors present at the time of the orientation. Last comes the implementation of the decision. This requires action. One tactical adage states that, 'Decisions without actions are pointless. Actions without decisions are reckless.' Then, because we hope that our actions will have changed the situation, the cycle begins anew. The cycle continues to repeat itself throughout a tactical operation.

"The adversary who can consistently go through Boyd's Cycle faster than the other gains a tremendous advantage. By the time the slower adversary reacts, the faster one is doing something different and the action becomes ineffective. With each cycle, the slower party's action is ineffective by a larger and larger margin. The aggregate resolution of these episodes will eventually determine the outcome of the conflict. For example, as long as the actions of the authorities continue to prove successful, a suspect will remain in a reactive posture, while the commander maintains the freedom to act. No matter what the suspect desperately strives to accomplish, every action becomes less useful than the preceding one. As a result, the suspect falls farther and farther behind. This demonstrates that the initiative follows the faster adversary [meaning you can control the encounter by being faster than the other guy]."

A simplified OODA situation

You are standing on the corner at 11 pm waiting for a bus when you see (Observe) to your right a couple of hoodlum types walking hard toward you. Your heart rate accelerates instantly and your brain kicks into survival mode. They are still about 50 feet away as you make a quick study of them and your environment (Orient): There is a bus stop bench next to you, between you and the two hoods, a two-lane street two steps to your front, and a building 10 feet to your left. To free your hands, you set your bag on the bench and stand ready, eyeing the pair as they approach.

One of them walks boldly up to you, stopping about five feet away on the same side of the bench as you, and the other stops on the other side (Orient again). "A good night for you to die, man," the closest one says.

You keep a neutral face as your brain formulates a plan (Decide): The instant he moves, you are going to slam your fist into his throat and then dash across the street to a grocery before the other can come around the bench.

"They call me Blademan," the closest one snarls, reaching under his coat. But before he can withdraw his hand, you lunge forward, jamming his arm against his chest with your left hand, and driving a hard, right cross into his Adam's apple (Act). As he falls across the bench, you do a fast about-face and bolt across the street toward the convenience store.

Understand that as you go through your OODA loop, the hoodlums are going through theirs. Up to the point where you punched the closest man, the hoods had Observed you, Oriented themselves to you, and Decided what to do. But just as the closest one started to Act on his decision, you thumped his neck. As he crumpled across the bench, the second hood was forced to start another OODA loop. He Observed what you did to his buddy, Oriented himself to you dashing across the street, and Decided whether he should stay with his injured friend or pursue you. If the sudden change in events surprised and alarmed him to any great extent, it will slow his Decision process so that you might make it all the way to the phone to call 9-1-1 before he can Decide how to Act, and escape into the night with his gagging friend.

A critical part of using Boyd's cycle is to understand the importance of the observation, orientation and decision phases. Most martial artists spend their time honing the action phase, that is, they train hard to make their punches and kicks formidable weapons. But as noted earlier, the best weapons are of no use if you can't bring them into play, if you can't make them work during a window of opportunity. To do so, it's vital that you streamline the first three stages of the OODA loop to pass through them as quickly as possible.

Let's look at an important training method that has been used in the military and various sports activities for a long time: To best prepare for the event, you must mimic the activity as closely as possible in your training. You still need to train your physical techniques - speed, power and precise body mechanics - but in a way they become almost secondary to the importance of getting "experience" from training as realistically as possible.

You and OODA

There are two issues you need to cover in training. The first is to reduce the time you spend in the OODA loop, or minimize the number of loops needed before you achieve your goal. Know that the longer you spend in the loop, the more time your opponent has to score a point in a sparring session or to ram a knife in your gut in a violent assault. It's only through sound training that you greatly reduce the chance of these undesirable things happening. On the flip side, you want to do everything you can to make your opponent waste time having to deal with his OODA loops.

Him slow, you fast: a winning combination.

Experience: real and manufactured

When you are somewhat conditioned to the stress and adrenaline rush of real violence, your brain takes less time to observe, orient and decide in the OODA loop because it's done it before under similar conditions. It draws on your previous experience to help provide you with fast solutions and then moves you quickly into the action phase for your fast response. It would be nice if you never had to face an attack that you hadn't trained for, but we all know that life doesn't work that way. Therefore, it's important to train for every possibility. Though there is no equivalent to actual, real fighting experience, good, realistic training is as close as you can get.

Make your training realistic In his book *Martial Arts America,* Bob Orlando wrote: "Begin by accepting the fact that all training is based on the *simulation* of reality. The operative word here is 'simulation.'" We agree. Never mistake your training for the real thing, but do strive to mimic it as closely as possible. For example, train occasionally in your heavy shoes and tight jeans. Train without hand and foot pads. Train in the alleyway behind your school or in a cramped, junk-filled basement. Put pads on a partner so you can land full-contact kicks and punches as he relentlessly stalks you.

If you want to compete, and it's your first time, go to one or two tournaments first as a spectator to get a feel for them, especially the energy and atmosphere. Then try to simulate those conditions in your training as closely and as often as possible. You might organize a crowd of parents and friends and encourage them to cheer and make noise. Your teacher should serve as the announcer and referee as you go through all the protocols that exist in a real tournament. After performing, analyze what you did well and what needs improvement. Then when you do enter a tournament, it will be less intimidating because your training has conditioned your brain to similar stimuli that exists in real matches. As a result, your trips through the OODA loop will be considerably smoother than had you not trained in this fashion.

Demeere didn't prepare this way for his first full-contact tournament. His teacher knew little of planning for competition, so Demeere's preparation consisted of going all-out against a few classmates the day before the event. Though he had attended one or two competitions before, he still didn't know entirely what to expect. Compounding the problem was that he wasn't given time to warm-up prior to his first fight, which is vital to prepare the muscles and tendons of the legs to deliver full-contact blows and block the opponent's full-contact leg kicks. Nonetheless, he charged in "like a maniac." He managed to win on a technical knockout, but a few minutes later, as he rested at the sidelines, his cold legs throbbed with excruciating pain, and his shinbones were red and swollen from all the leg kicks he had slammed into his opponent.

He had to fight again an hour later, and although he had time to warm-up, he couldn't because his legs were in such agony. The fight turned quickly into a brawl, one that Demeere has no recollection of even today. His coach said that he seemed to go berserk, delivering three attacks for every one he received. When he and his opponent crashed to the floor, Demeere continued fighting (a violation of the rules), and the referee had to pull him off his opponent several times. He did win the match, though the entire crowd booed him as he left the fighting area.

Demeere's lack of memory of the fight is most likely a result of his stress-induced accelerated heart rate, probably in the range of 175 beats per minute. (A stress-induced heart rate isn't the same as an accelerated rate from sparring or jogging.) His high heart rate and lack of experience with such high caliber competition caused his brain to be unable to process and remember details. Even worse was that the stress of being unprepared prevented him from fighting well. Though Demeere did win second place, he had probably gotten stuck somewhere around the orient and decide phases of the OODA loop, so that virtually all of his technical skills deserted him, leaving only an animalistic and out-of-control fighting spirit.

Since Demeere is an analytical fighter, the experience wasn't wasted on him; he realized a need for specific training. He knew that his technical and physical attributes were fine, but it was the lack of mental and psychological preparation for the event that made his performance so poor.

Self-defense training   Role playing works well for self-defense training. Most people who have been attacked and fought well agree that it wasn't necessarily technique that saved the day for them, but rather their mental commitment. There are no referees in the street; it's just you and the big ape with bulging veins in his forehead. If you can't overcome the stress response and if you can't function with an accelerated heart rate, the benefactor of your life insurance plan will be wearing a big smile and driving a fine new car. Though it will always be frightening and stressful to face an adversary bent on rearranging your facial features, it's possible to function well under stress if you have trained for it. Here are a few training ideas for your workouts. Feel free to make up more scenarios.

- Start out slowly with a training partner who acts like a loud, drunken idiot looking for a fight. Focus on keeping him at a safe distance, watching his movements and being aware of objects and obstacles in your environment. Understand that there is nothing physical going on at this stage. The idea is for you to get a *feel* for a verbally aggressive person in your face and to practice observing and orientating yourself to him. Practice two or three different scenarios.

- Once you are fairly comfortable with scenarios where your training partner is loud and obnoxious, begin to add a physical element to each new one: In the next scenario, he continues to yell and curse (while you observe and orient yourself), then physically pushes you (you quickly decide how to respond and then act on it). You knock aside his hands. In the next one, he grabs your shirt or arm, and you escape from the hold. In the last scenario, he punches and kicks, and you block and counter. Through all the scenarios, which have gotten progressively more physical, he keeps up the verbal tirade. If you aren't careful, you will find that his threats and shouting can interfere with your OODA looping.

Save the last scenario, the punching or kicking attack, until you are ready for the greater intensity, which could take several workouts. The basis of this type of training is to develop and condition yourself mentally and physically. Training progressively provides your brain with experience to deal with stress and the specifics of real violence. It also educates your mind to the different OODA loops that occur in a violent encounter and helps you move through them quickly. Though the specific details of a real situation might be different than in your training, your brain will recognize the conditions - stress, adrenaline, verbal aggression, attempts to blindside you - so you will be less surprised, thus freeing your brain to focus quickly on the action phase of OODA.

Be careful with the realism You need to tread carefully with this training. It's easy to get carried away, especially when you aren't used to it. Early on in co-author Christensen's police career, he introduced a more intense defensive tactics program to a new group of police rookies. Greater force was encouraged, and techniques were executed close to all-out. While it was a good idea on paper, Christensen skipped the phase where the recruits started slowly and progressively, but instead had them jump right into the fray. The new program came to a screeching halt two weeks later after Christensen was called before a deputy chief to explain why a clock and several framed pictures on the adjoining wall in the district attorney's office had been knocked down and broken, why one of the professional actors hired to help in the scenario had been choked out, and why a recruit had to be whisked away by ambulance to get stitches in his face.

It's important to start slowly and increase the intensity by small increments. It's also a good idea to have a third person monitor the drill to ensure that no one gets hurt. Should he see one participant get into trouble, he stops the drill instantly. An available first aid kit is a good idea, too. Seriously.

Some people, especially the so-called "traditional" martial artists, tend to disparage this type of training. They feel their training methods, ones inherited from centuries ago, are more than sufficient to carry them through any violent situation in the mean streets. Though there is truth in that idea for some people, it's not everyone's truth. Some people are born with a strong warrior spirit and tend to become superior fighters when trained in the ancient ways. Others, however, benefit more from scenario training, a dynamic tool that helps them overcome their anxieties, break through psychological barriers, and shoot through their OODA loops like a well-greased piece of machinery. Even for people with experience, it can be worthwhile.

On one occasion, Demeere was teaching a self-defense course and selected a tall, strong participant for a specific scenario. Playing the role of the antagonist, Demeere began verbally insulting the man, increasing the intensity of his verbal tirade to a point where he physically attacked the student. The man tried to hold Demeere back and even pushed him once, all the while Demeere cuffed his face with what appeared to be ineffective slaps. After the scenario ended, Demeere asked the man and the other participants what was wrong with what they had just witnessed. When no one knew the answer, Demeere opened his hand to reveal a small folding knife he had taken out of his pocket during the scenario. Not one person had seen him do it. His slap-like attacks were actually cuts and stabs at specific targets on the man, simulated of course, but only because Demeere had not opened the knife. The students' lack of familiarity with the verbal aggression and the stress it causes, kept them from seeing a crucial factor in the brief encounter. All had failed the observation phase of OODA. The good news, and the purpose behind Demeere's lesson, was that from that point on everyone paid close attention to what his hands were doing.

Force him into the OODA loop

When practicing scenario training, or any type of realistic drills, your objective is to reduce your time in Boyd's cycle, since the longer there, the slower you are to respond. Conversely, you want to do all that you can to make your opponent spend lots of time in the loop, to make it difficult, even impossible, for him to defend or attack you. If you can continue to force him into the cycle, he has to think about what he needs to do, all the while you are pressing forward with your attack. Your goal is to present him with numerous signals, all at once or in succession. You want to continuously force him into the first stages of the loop. That way whatever action he does decide upon will inevitably fail because his action will be based on information that is no longer current. He is forced continuously to try to catch up, but he can't because you remain in his face.

As you recall in the earlier scenario where Blademan tried to attack you, you moved quickly through OODA and jammed his arm and punched his Adam's apple. His OODA was out the window, as he was too busy writhing on the ground and clawing at what felt like a cement truck lodged in his throat. His buddy, though, was starting a new OODA based on the turn of events. He observed your action and oriented himself to where he stood behind the bus bench. When you took off across the street, he decided to help his buddy get out of there. But let's add something new.

Say when Blademan fell to the ground, his knife dropped from his hand. Both you and his buddy observe the weapon and the two of you orient yourself to it. The other guy is farther away from it than you. While he is trying to decide if he should run or leap over the bench to get the weapon, you decide and act first by picking it up. Now the guy behind the bench has to begin another OODA: He observes you pick it up; he orients himself to you and the new threat, he decides whether to fight you or flee, but before he can act, you dash off across the street. Again he starts a new OODA: He observes you run off; he feels comfortable in his orientation to you and the expanding distance from you; he decides to pick up Blademan and skitter off into the night.

Even in this simple scenario, Blademan's buddy was kept busy OODA looping. Should you have stayed and fought him (it was much smarter that you fled), you would have had lots of timing opportunities because of his occupied brain.

Though we needed nearly half a page to explain the different OODA loops Blademan's partner was making, in reality each four-part loop takes a second or two to complete. While this might seem fast, a lot can happen in a second or two. Some well-trained fighters can throw multiple blows in a second. This is bad news if it's you going, "Uhhh?" to a change in the scenario, but good news if it's you forcing your adversary into the loops.

Here are a few ways to force your opponent back into the OODA loop.

- **Use an auditory stimulus:** Launch your attack while he is in mid-sentence. Shout loudly as you attack.

As the man speaks . . . .

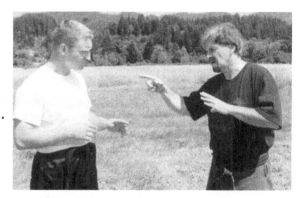

hit him in mid sentence.

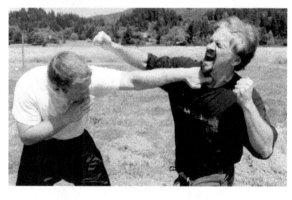

- **Don't remain static**   Use footwork to confuse your opponent by forcing him to continuously analyze your movement patterns and range changes, all of which slows his ability to attack you.

• **Use natural movements as set-ups for an attack:** Learn to talk with your hands like a bad actor portraying a gangster so that your opponent becomes conditioned to seeing them in his space. Then when a timing moment occurs, launch your attack from one of the gestures, a movement that will be hard for him to detect.

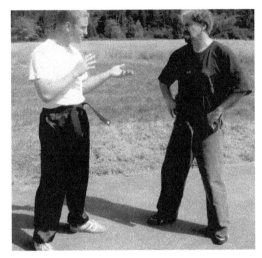

Use your hands as you talk to camouflage your attack.

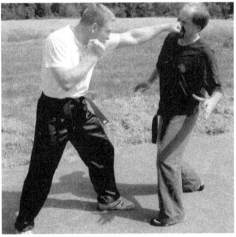

• **Start with a fast attack to the eyes** This forces him to instinctively blink or pull his head away. Immediately follow with a hard blow of some kind, or move away at an angle to force him to reorient himself to where you are. When the hit is timed well, it feels to the opponent as if he had time only to dodge that first attack before you hit him with another. When you move away at an angle, he has to find you with pained eyes, which gives you all kinds of time to flee or hit him again.

- **Strike first in a street confrontation.** When you connect first, you daze your adversary or at least distract him with pain. By taking the initiative, you become, in effect, faster than him by having slowed his ability to go through the OODA loop, especially the orientation part of the cycle. Once you have the advantage over your opponent, it becomes increasingly more difficult for him to recover, especially if you continue to rain blows on him. (You should research your local laws since preemptive strikes are not always a legal option.)

- **Strike first in competition.** This is usually an effective way to start a match because it immediately forces your opponent into a new OODA loop.

- **Don't limit yourself to single techniques.** It's usually more effective to use continuous combinations to overwhelm your opponent. A bombardment of blows puts more on his plate, hopefully more than he can chew, er, block. Each explosive combination presents new information that forces him back into the observation phase of the loop. This keeps him on the defensive, with no other choice than to try and limit the damage he receives. This is a powerful fighting principle that allows you to hit first and almost at will, since it's virtually impossible to block all the attacks of a good combination.

The concept of the OODA loop is a marvelous one that we reference often throughout this book. Actually, warriors have used OODA since early cavemen figured out that bashing Og in the head with a T-Rex bone was a good way to steal his food and get his woman. Move forward a few hundred thousand years and we are at Pearl Harbor and the Day of Infamy. Taken by total surprise, the American military was stuck in the observation, orientation and decision phases for what must have felt like ages before they began to return fire at the Japanese planes.

It's interesting to note that OODA not only works to provide timing advantages in a fight, it's used in other sporting activities to confuse opponents, it's used by corporations in the dog-eat-dog world of big business, and it's used in Iraq by the military as we pen this book. Indeed, the OODA loop concept was used in the past and continues to be used today in all areas of life.

OODA loop. Fun to say, important to master, and so effective to use against your opponent.

Types of reactions

Simply stated, an untrained person is more likely to react to a surprise stimulus in an uncontrollable and erratic manner, while a trained person is more likely to react with finesse and close to an ideal response. The better you understand the types of reactions the more you are able to tailor your training so that *you* can use them, rather than having them used against you. Let's look at the different types.

Reflexes

Reflex actions are your body's way of using shortcuts. In previous paragraphs, we talked about how the brain receives information, analyzes it and then reacts to it, steps that take but a fraction of a second. However, sometimes even that isn't fast enough. Reflexes happen when your body receives a stimulus that it interprets as dangerous. The reaction that follows - startle, muscle tensing, inhalation of breath, or a squeal - occurs before the stimulus reaches the brain. It's a primal reaction that comes from the spine. It's similar to when the doctor taps your knee and your leg pops up a little. Your brain didn't order the action; it's automatic, a short cut. The action is typically a singular movement: a jerk of the hand, a contraction of the muscles, or a blink of the eyes. The reflex system exists because there are certain dangers in the world that if you were to wait on your brain to go through the OODA loop, you are going to get hurt. For example:

- When you accidentally place your hand on a hot stove, you yank it back before your brain receives a signal that it's being barbequed.

- When something flies at your face and your eyes automatically close.

- When you hear a sudden, loud sound and your muscles contract causing you to jump.

Instinctive actions   Although the line between instinctive reactions and reflexes is sometimes blurred, here is a good, working definition: Instinctive actions are generally a sequence of movements to avoid a specific danger or to adapt to a change in the environment. Each action looked at separately isn't useful in and of itself. But when you look at them as a whole, they lead to an action that preserves your life. Here is an example.

One night in his teens, co-author Demeere was walking home from a party when he heard the distinct sound of a car's screeching tires directly behind him. He spun around just in time to see a sedan miss a turn and go into a skid. The driver, later to be found drunk, overcompensated and put the 3000-pound car into a collision course with young Demeere. Though it must have been a very fast move, Demeere remembers leaping in slow motion, a move he says that wasn't flashy like those of a movie hero's, but was more like a cross between a running kangaroo and a jumping chicken. There was no time to think about good form; it was all about pure survival instinct. The car did miss him, but only by a few inches.

Here are more examples of instincts in action:

- Two men are fighting and Man A begins to get the upper hand. When Man B is knocked to the floor he realizes he is overpowered, so he covers his head and curls his body into a fetal position, an instinctive attempt to minimize damage. He remains like that until the assault stops.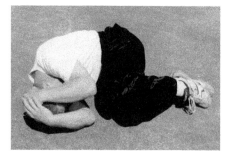

- Demeere once witnessed a junkie running into three of his drug dealers at the wrong time. He must have owed them money because as soon as they saw him, they began making verbal threats. The junkie stepped back, dropped to the ground, and made placating gestures, all the while avoiding eye contact with them. His was a classic instinctive gesture of submission, since a downed opponent is in principle less of a threat than a standing one.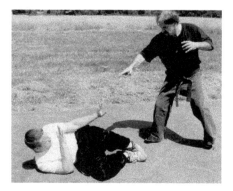

Trained responses   Instinct and reflex actions are seemingly arbitrary responses to specific situations, while trained responses are an entirely different animal. In the context of self-defense and martial arts, trained responses are actions or reactions that you specifically ingrain into your mind and body through your training. You determine what the best response is for a specific or general situation, say, a lead jab to the head, and then you drill in that response. Your goal is to do it so many times in a variety of ways - different attackers, slow and fast attacks, low lighting, on an uneven surface, on a cluttered floor - that your response becomes instinctual. As soon as you see that jab coming at you, or an attack that is similar, your trained response is there for you.

There are several ways to work your drills. Typically, a martial artist learns a specific technique and then practices it repetitiously. Sometimes this works, sometimes it doesn't, or it's less effective than it could be. An important factor here, and a logical one often missed by fighters, is to consider if the specific defense being drilled actually works well against the attack you are facing. For example, if you train to fire off a high roundhouse kick against an attacker's jab, chances are he will hit you first, since his technique has less distance to travel to its target. Logical? Yes. But it's one lost on many fighters.

A problem arises, however, and it's a common one, is that while a fighter knows a response won't work on a subconscious level, his conscious mind tricks him into believing that it will. Should a real confrontation happen, there is a high likelihood that he will experience a conflicting set of mental commands and freeze, or at the very least, proceed slowly. This is because part of his brain says to do the roundhouse kick, while another part says, "That ain't gonna work, big boy. You should just move your head out of the way." While his brain is busy resolving this conflict, trapped in the decision phase of OODA, the jab smears his nose across his face.

The quality of the technique you drill into memory is also critical. *Quality* is the operative word here. As the saying goes: Garbage in, garbage out. When you face a meany on the street or a skilled competitor in the ring, clearly you don't want garbage coming out. Work diligently to understand your techniques; understand in what situations they are used; understand their limitations; understand their strengths.

Consider forms training. A student performs the techniques a certain way - exaggerated and often made prettier or altered to hide their meaning - but they are executed differently when applied against a live opponent in drills and sparring. Now, should that student get into a real fight and start to use one of the kata techniques, his subconscious tells him that the move won't work, or it's iffy, or it has to be modified someway. This leads to confusion and most likely defeat.

Early in his martial arts career, co-author Christensen studied two fighting styles that he now refers to as "robot karate." Both employed stiff punching and kicking techniques, and blocks that were rigid, regimented and totally unrealistic. Being new to the arts and having little fighting experience, Christensen accepted the teachings as the gospel truth. All of the students did then, because karate in the mid '60s was straight from Korea and Japan, so new in this country that few questioned its doctrines. Three years after he began training, Christensen found himself patrolling the war-torn streets, bars and brothels of Saigon, Vietnam as a military policeman. There were few days when he didn't get into a scuffle or an all-out fight. As such, it didn't take long for him to catch on that his robot karate - deep stances, step-over reverse punches, rising blocks, and high-chambered kicks - were not working for him. While he had tremendous power, his ingrained movements were so regimented that it was difficult to apply the techniques when someone was resisting arrest violently or simply trying to take his head off.

Although his 14-hour work shifts didn't allow time for training, he managed to modify a few basic techniques, tested them on the street, and survived the rest of his time in Vietnam. Upon returning home, and up to this day, Christensen has concentrated solely on street-oriented, realistic fighting techniques.

Natural blocks

All blocks should be structured to incorporate natural and instinctual reactions or reflexes, because the more natural they are, the faster they are. Instincts aren't set in stone. If you perform an instinctual reaction and it fails to protect you, your brain will often try to suppress or permanently inhibit it and then try to find one that does work. In the same way, if you do manage to protect yourself, your brain will ingrain that reaction more deeply, making it more likely to become an automatic response. Unfortunately, these responses are generally geared at avoiding danger (defense), not at putting an end to it (offense).

Cross arms block   Consider a natural reaction to a threat where you quickly cross your arms in front of your face. This is an instinctual and universal response (often accompanied with a squeal and a plea, "Don't hurt me.") to a sudden attack coming toward your head. But it's a passive one. The block alone doesn't allow you to counter your attacker, so all he has to do is throw a second blow under your arms.

Let's look at some ideas with which you can experiment with a partner to see how you can turn the crossing hands into a timing moment to launch a nasty counter. Let's make the attack the reverse punch and make crossing your hands in front of your face the defense. Here are some things you can do just with this simple, instinctual reaction. Notice how each response sets up a timing moment. Sometimes your attacker's fist will impact your wrists or forearms, and that is okay because you can still flow into a follow-up.

- Cross your hands to cover your face and duck your head. Duck straight down or to the left or right side as you lean forward slightly to absorb the impact. Immediately counter with blows to the body or execute a takedown.

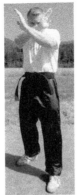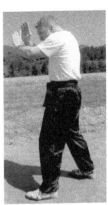

Cross block from the front and from the side

- As you cross your arms, step to the right or left of the punch. This places you in a good position to seize the opportunity to strike, kick or execute a throw.

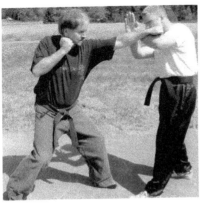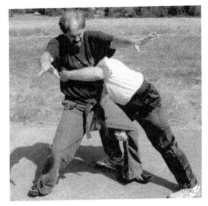

Cross block your opponent's jab and then shoot in for a takedown.

- Cross your arms and step backwards diagonally. As the punch glances off your arms, grab the attacking arm and pull at it with all your bodyweight as you move back. Pull him to the floor, into a table edge, or into your knee strike.

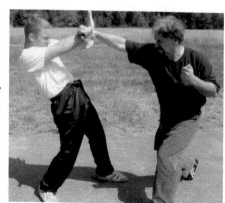

Cross block the reverse punch.

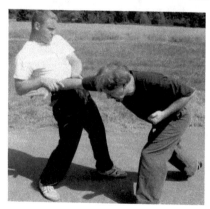

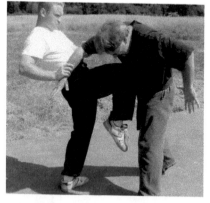

Grab his punching arm and pull him into a knee strike.

- Cross your arms and step sideways to your left or right, and pivot your body so you are sideways to your opponent. As you do, grab or control his punching arm with your rear hand and backfist him with your closest one.

- Cross your hands in such away that one hand slaps the incoming punch to the side as it moves up to save your face. Lean slightly away from the attack, placing your weight on your rear leg. Use the other leg to whip in a quick kick to the stomach, knee or groin.

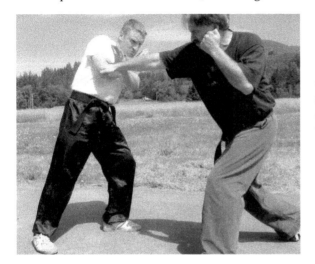

Cross block and sweep the punch away as you lean to the side.

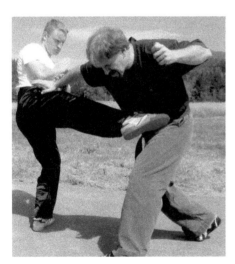 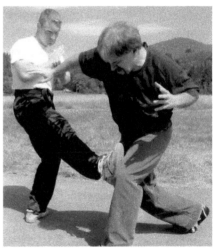

Snap a rear-leg kick into the groin (not pictured), the abdomen (or knee.

Practice 1 to 2 sets of 10 reps of each technique on both sides.

Use your creativity to find even more variations of using the natural reaction of protecting your face and flowing smoothly into a vicious counter. Once you feel comfortable with blocking and then hitting, experiment with simultaneous blocking and countering. If you train on these techniques 30 minutes a day, everyday for two weeks, you will discover two happy findings. First, is their versatility. The five techniques listed above were just made up quickly to include here. Should you spend 10 minutes playing with just one of them, four or five other variations will occur to you, all of which offer perfect timing moments. Secondly, after those two weeks of training, compare your speed with these new, yet natural, techniques against other defensive moves you have learned in your art. You might find to your amazement, as have other fighters, that you can execute these moves just as fast as the other blocks you have been doing for years.

The reason for your accelerated learning curve and the high quality of your performance is the instinctual nature of the defense. You aren't training your subconscious mind to do something entirely new and awkward, but rather you are working with an existing reaction, one your mind knows instinctually will work. You begin with a natural movement and then tweak it a little to improve it even more. In the end, you own a versatile and extremely fast technique that gives you a definite timing advantage over your opponent. It's all about simplicity, which is what fighting techniques should be about.

More instinctual defensive actions   Another example of young Christensen's gullibility early on was his acceptance of his style's backfist defense. Here is how it worked, or how it was supposed to have worked. Say you are in a left-leg forward fighting stance when your opponent launches a left backfist. To block, you would lift up your left arm, your fist about head high, palm-side toward you, and move it toward the attack. To give your arm support, you would place your right palm on your left forearm. Timing wise, the instant you recognized the hint of a backfist, you were supposed to step in and slam your supported forearm against his, just as it was beginning its launch. The concept was based on the fact that the attacker's arm is weakest at its origin, before it begins to extend toward the target.

Sounds good on paper, but putting it into play was another story. Other than an extremely fast veteran fighter doing it against a new student 30 minutes into his first lesson, it's impossible to execute. The timing doesn't work because the backfist is a naturally fast technique, with some fighters possessing a lightening-quick strike that is nearly imperceptible. So, by the time you see the launch of the backfist and process through the OODA loop, the attacker's fist is just inches from your nose, if not two or three inches *into* your nose.

Christensen noted that when his classmates sparred, they didn't respond to a backfist with the way-too-slow block they had all been taught, but rather lifted their lead arms toward the attack and ducked their heads a little. This natural reaction wasn't fancy, but it worked. When Christensen began teaching, he eliminated the old backfist block, which no one missed because no one was using it, anyway, and replaced it with a move where the blocker raises his forearm diagonally, leans his body back slightly and tilts his head a little to the side. It's a fast, effective block that stops or slows the blow, shields the head, and creates opportunities to execute well-timed counters.

Another example of what seemed to be a good idea but then mostly failed in reality occurred when Christensen was on the police department. Although officers had carried the straight baton (a 24-inch nightstick made of wood, aluminum or some kind of space-age material) for years, mostly without complaint, an administrator decided to change everyone's baton to the side-handled one, a baton that is 24 inches in length with a handle protruding from the side about 1/3 of the way from one end. Its creator based the weapon's design on the tonfa, an old Okinawan weapon. By gripping the side handle, one can deliver several more pounds of thrust than with the straight baton, and an incredible amount of force when whipping the weapon into the kneecap of a hapless criminal. The problem is that it's an unnatural action, especially under stress.

Give a straight baton to a toddler and he whacks the kitty's head with natural form and grace. Give a cop four to eight hours training with a side-handled baton, and toward the end of the session he looks good in the air and on a practice dummy. But it's a whole different story when some ex-con with weight-trained muscles and tattoos on his face wants some payback. Under stress, many officers resorted to using the side-handled baton like a regular straight one, or if they did try to whip it, they failed to use the right body mechanics, which made their blows ineffectual. Of those officers who were effective with the side-handled baton, most were martial artists who spent extra time training with it.

The moral of the story is that most often it's best to remain with a technique or weapon that is grounded in natural movements and natural reactions. You will never be optimally fast or have superb timing when your muscles have to perform awkwardly and your brain has to struggle though unnatural movements. Timing moments are more easily exploited when you react quickly and naturally.

A final thought on reflexes and instinctual actions

Reflexes and instinctual reactions play an important role in the martial arts. While both can be triggered when fighting in the street or in the ring, the difference is that reflexes are hard to alter because the brain isn't involved in them. Reflexes are triggered directly from the spinal chord. However, understanding how they work and then trying consciously to avoid them from happening can overcome some reflexes. For example, winking or closing the eyes is a reflexive action to a sudden threat at your face, an action seen typically in new students. But after training for a while, they become conditioned to the attack, and are able to suppress the reflex enough to keep their eyes open and execute their counter technique. The reflex is still there and can still be triggered, but they have learned to block it to some degree.

Instinctual actions can be tweaked a little or a lot depending on how much quality training you put in. You saw how you can alter the instinctual action of crossing your hands in front of your face to make the movement applicable in a fight. The key to making these reactions work for self-defense is to stay close to their nature. Any tweaking you do should not alter the reaction to such a degree that it no longer resembles its original form.

Hick's Law

A fox was boasting to a cat of its clever devices for escaping its enemies. "I have a whole bag of tricks," he said, "which contains a hundred ways of escaping my enemies."

"I have only one," said the cat. "But I can generally manage with that."

Just at that moment they heard the cry of a pack of hounds coming towards them, and the cat immediately scampered up a tree and hid herself in the boughs. "This is my plan," said the Cat. "What are you going to do?"

The Fox thought first of one way, then of another, and while he was debating the hounds came nearer and nearer, and at last the fox in his confusion was caught up by the hounds and soon killed by the huntsmen. The cat that had been looking on, said, "Better one safe way than a hundred on which you cannot reckon."

Allow us to get a little academic for a moment and talk about something called Hick's Law, a principle developed in the 1950s that continues to be studied to this day. It's one every martial artist needs to understand. We are going to skip the complex aspects and focus instead on that part that is most relevant to timing.

A technical definition

Hick's Law states that reaction time increases approximately 150 milliseconds when the response option (technique) increases from one to two. This means that a person's reaction time increases proportionally when the number of skills in a system increases. This is because more time is required to process, select and organize the appropriate response to a threat. Therefore, according to Hicks, when milliseconds can mean the difference between life and death, a system consisting of a small number of techniques increases the defender's chance of survival.

Our definition

We define Hick's Law to mean that the more choices you have to complete a specific task, the longer it takes you to choose one. So, if you trained on 10 different defenses against a front kick, it's likely that kick will land in your gut before you can select one with which to defend yourself.

How Christensen applied Hick's Law without knowing it

When Christensen began training in a traditional Korean style in 1965, he learned virtually a different block for every kick. A sidekick was blocked this way and a roundhouse kick was blocked that way. That was fine until he progressed in rank and trained with people who could kick with great speed and deception. The concept didn't work as well then because it was difficult, sometimes impossible, to determine which kick the advance fighter was executing until it landed with a thud.

When Christensen began teaching, and had yet to hear of Hick's Law, he eliminated all the blocks but one, a simple one that could be applied to a variety of kicks. With just a minor adjustment in body angle or a slight step to one side or the other, this one, lonesome block stops or deflects most kicks. This makes for faster blocking and a more solid defense because there is no time spent deciding which block to use. When a kick is launched, there is just one response.

Hick's Law and our frontline warriors

Law enforcement and the military both incorporate Hick's Law in their training to minimize or avoid time-wasting steps that place the soldier or police officer at risk. Consisting of only a handful of techniques, their self-defense programs appear quite limited compared to what most martial arts schools offer. And it's true: Hand-to-hand training, with or without weapons (firearms excluded), is given very little training time when compared to other necessary skills, such as how to enter a building in which there are suspected terrorists or how to search prisoners for weapons, tasks of crucial importance to professionals working in life and death situations. Soldiers simply don't have the time to spend hours each day training to defend against a straight punch. Nor do they need to. When faced with violence, they operate under different rules than nonmilitary people. An enemy in a war zone is more likely to get shot than punched, especially if the soldier has a choice between using his weapon and using unarmed techniques. However, when he does have to use empty-hand techniques, the soldier uses a simple movement that dispatches the threat quickly.

Is less best for the street?

For those wanting effective self-defense without spending years of continuous study, a simple set of techniques is arguably more than enough to handle most street confrontations. For the "average" street altercation, you don't need to be a martial arts master. With a limited set of tools, good training and the right mind-set, you have a better than good chance of reigning victorious. Limiting your arsenal to only a few techniques gives you a definite speed advantage and a good ability to seize a timing moment.

The martial arts, however, offer a complete system of unarmed combat techniques, focusing mostly on the fight itself. Much more than law enforcement and the military, modern martial artists continuously explore their systems, examining what is useful in other systems and styles, and always striving to develop new techniques or subtle variations on old ones.

The other side of the argument

Is it possible to simplify your actions in a fight to the extent that you oversimplify them? How few techniques are too few at the risk of being unable to respond to the most common types of attacks? What might happen should you face an experienced street fighter who knows a variety of techniques? Will your handful of techniques be sufficient to deal with him? What will you do should your technique miss or fail to have the desired effect? These are important questions that might be harder to answer than first realized.

We feel Hick's Law is an important concept but it needs to be used wisely and constructively. If you are interested in pure self-defense, have limited time to train and want to keep things simple and effective, then you want to apply Hick's Law to your training. But if you want to progress beyond that and explore the fighting arts in greater detail, you will naturally want to practice a greater number of techniques. You still want to apply Hick's Law in various phases of your continuous study, but most likely you will study far more techniques than the soldier or police officer.

One must tread carefully when simplifying things because sometimes you need more than just a few techniques. Your initial move might have missed or glanced off your attacker, or his solid block might have forced you to start over. Or the situation might be such that another, perhaps more difficult technique is more appropriate. Consider these situations:

- Demeere was once involved in a brawl with two adversaries where he quickly doubled over the closest one with a hard blow to his stomach. The next attacker had positioned himself poorly by standing right behind the first one, though the second man didn't think about this until Demeere's high roundhouse kick flew over his bent-over buddy and slammed into the side of his very surprised face.

- On another occasion Demeere had to throw a violent drunk out of a bar in his duties as a bouncer. When the man attacked, Demeere first threw the drunk to the floor, scooted around behind and inserted his index fingers into the corners of the man's mouth, "fish-hooking" him into a restraint hold. That worked, but only a little, so Demeere switched to a tai chi chuan grappling technique to flip him onto the floor and get control of him. At that point, two of the drunk's friends grabbed Demeere's arms, which he quickly shook off, but in so doing lost contact of the drunk. This time Demeere grabbed the guy in a muay Thai clinch and escorted him out the door.

- Once in competition, Demeere was having trouble closing the gap on a strong and skilled opponent without getting hit. Changing tactics, Demeere took two quick steps and jumped on top of his opponent, then threw a fast and hard punch into the man's surprised face, a move that changed the rhythm of the sparring session to his advantage.

- Once when Christensen was working patrol, he was called to a church to help other police officers who were trying to take a Taiwanese muay Thai fighter into custody. Earlier, the man, who doctors later determined to be quite insane, had walked into a church service from a freezing winter storm, shirtless and shoeless, ran over to the minister at the front of the congregation, and kicked him in the face, knocking the man down. The fighter then found his way to the attic where he lay down and waited for the police. The first two officers on the scene were quickly knocked back with kicks to their faces. When Christensen arrived at the scene, he recalls trying not to laugh at one of the officers who had a perfect mud footprint across his forehead. Christensen suggested they change tactics and grab hold of one side of an old, full-sized mattress lying in a corner of the attic. On Christensen's count of three, they rushed toward the muay Thai man with their huge shield, and slammed the mattress down on the fighter before he could get to his feet. As two officers sat on the mattress, the other two applied restraints to the ankles extending from one end and handcuffs to the wrists extending from the other.

Now, we aren't boasting here about our fighting successes or claiming that these were the best techniques, though they did work to end each problem, which is the bottom line. They definitely weren't techniques taught in a basic self-defense class. Demeere's techniques took a lot of time and training to gain proficiency in because they are more complex than basic ones. His high roundhouse kick that went over one man's head and into the face of another is hardly the wisest move in a self-defense situation, but rather the stuff of a Jackie Chan movie. Yet it worked that one time. Christensen's story is a prime example of improvising in ways that go well beyond basic techniques. Blindly following Hick's Law would have had him going at that muay Thai fighter using only one or two select punches and kicks. That would have meant one heck of a fight, with a real possibility of serious injury to one or both of them. However, with a little creativity he managed to get the man into custody without either of them receiving a scratch.

The fact that we had a wider range of options at our disposal in these incidents than Hick's law would dictate, allowed us to accomplish our tasks. But please don't read into this that you should learn as many techniques as possible. We believe that both extremes are to be avoided: too many techniques are as bad as too few (just ask the aforementioned fox. Actually, it's too late to ask him anything). You must find a balance between what you can achieve technically and what is to be expected should you have to defend yourself. It's a mistake to assume you will only fight incompetent beginners, and it's equally foolish to assume you will only face trained killers with dozens of notches carved in their revolver grips. The truth lies somewhere in the middle.

Hick's law is frequently misunderstood. Too often it's used to simplify just for simplification's sake, rather than to enhance the quality of a fighting curriculum. Don't look at the concept in a vacuum, but be open to other factors that have an influence on it: the complexity of the choices; the familiarity of the fighter with those choices; the fighter's confidence; and his tolerance to stress. All of these influence the time it takes to make a decision.

Influences Christensen and his police partner were searching a backyard for an armed hold-up man who had just robbed a liquor store. At one point the two officers separated. Christensen ran along side a solid wooden fence with a plan of going around the end of it and into the backyard, as his partner pulled himself up and partially over it, unaware the hold-up man was crouched on the side. The instant the officer's face appeared, the suspect fired a bullet into his mouth, ripping a pathway through his tongue and lodging next to his spine.

Christensen didn't see his partner get hit, though he heard a muffled shot, so muffled that he wasn't sure if it really was gunfire. He pushed through heavy branches of a walnut tree, suddenly coming face-to-face with the gunman who looked just as surprised as Christensen probably did. Christensen raised his weapon but then hesitated ever so briefly as a multitude of thoughts streaked across his brain: *Was that really a gunshot I heard? Is this the suspect? Does he fit the description? Is my partner okay? Will I get into trouble if I shoot him?* Though the thoughts passed at the speed of light, they took long enough that the suspect spun and fled. The barrage of thoughts caused Christensen to miss the window of opportunity.

A minute later, however, Christensen confronted the suspect again, and this time he saw a long-barreled revolver in the man's hand. The situation was no longer a complex one, as the presence of the gun made the decision easy. Christensen fired.

A friend of Demeere's, who used to work as a bouncer, began studying the martial arts as a child, studying a number of fighting disciplines well into his adulthood. Through his work, he has been exposed to countless violent encounters, some life threatening. He has relied on his punches from boxing, high kicks from traditional kung fu, leg kicks from muay Thai, joint locks from aikido, head butts from kali and elbow strikes from pentjak silat. Some were basic techniques, while others seemed to come straight out of a martial arts movie. While so many techniques from so many fighting arts might seem to contradict Hick's law, it doesn't. We use his example to show you how other factors can have an important influence on performance during an actual situation. Such as:

- If you are used to performing under the adrenaline stress of a real fight, you can pull off more complex techniques than if you aren't. Experience can make a difference.

- Your reaction time is slower when you see something from your peripheral vision than when you see it in plain sight. The sooner you see something, the more time you have to execute a technique, even an advanced one.

- If you are alert and mentally ready, you will react faster to an attack than when tired, drowsy, or not paying attention.

- If you train a technique consistently (thousands of times) under a variety of circumstances, you have a better chance of using it successfully in the street, even if it's not a basic technique.

The list goes on, but you can see that Hick's Law isn't written in stone. You need to see it in this larger context and also understand the factors that counter the effects of this law.

Our approach is pragmatic and simplistic, as yours should be. Your core techniques, the foundation of your fighting skills, should not revolve around fancy or flashy moves. Build a solid base but don't feel content once you have it in place: keep exploring new training methods and experimenting to get better at your basics. Add techniques and ideas, but only if you feel they are important to your overall theme. In other words, don't just collect techniques for no other reason than to stockpile. How large your repertoire becomes depends on your needs. That said, know that it's okay to play with a variety of techniques and ideas because your study of the fighting arts should also be fun and interesting. However, your real sweat and tears should come from drilling hard on your core techniques so that they are there for you in a fraction of a second, when a timing opportunity occurs.

Mental components

Even if you have highly-trained reflexes and train hard on a variety of drills, that doesn't translate necessarily into an ability to execute perfect timing. You need more than just the physical: You also need the right mind-set.

An Eastern approach

There is a concept in Japanese martial arts called Mushin, literally translated as "no-mind." There have been volumes written about it, but to define it in a few words....Mushin is a mental state in which your mind becomes detached from itself, so to speak. You no longer consciously think about what is going on, but rather let things happen by themselves. Small or even large things, such as the sound of a barking dog or a passing car, don't distract you. You know they are there and acknowledge their presence, but they don't dominate your attention. You are simply in the moment as your mind encompasses all things, while not focusing on any one. When unattached and not anticipating, your mind is open to whatever happens. However, when it focuses on one thing, it has become attached and you no longer have no-mind.

Say you are sparring with a fellow student who has a whip-like backfist. As the two of you stalk each other, you are ready mentally for his backfist, with a plan to block it and then counter with a – *Bam!* he just kicked you in the stomach. Okay, lucky shot. You stalk him again, ever so ready for that deadly backfist of his. When it comes, you are ready with a – *Bam!* he got you with a fast uppercut punch. Your opponent is scoring on you easily because your mind is focused on his backfist, thus allowing his other techniques to get you.

When you anticipate, you make a prediction and, to state the obvious, predictions either hit or miss. When you anticipate on one or two possibilities, you eliminate a host of others. Yes, sometimes it works, but should you be wrong, you might lose the street fight, the tournament, or your life.

Imagine that your mind is a mirror, reflecting everything it sees. It doesn't think about what it reflects, nor does it pass judgment. It only reflects. Mushin is a way to free your mind from the distractions and diversions conscious thinking brings. By allowing your mind to be free of distractions, you can react more naturally and more quickly to a timing moment.

Other examples of Mushin Though this might sound mystical and perhaps even esoteric, it really isn't. If you are a skilled typist and can type a letter, carry on a conversation, and watch television all at the same time, your act of typing is no-mind. When you run up a long set of stairs and your thoughts are focused on what you are going to do when you get to the top, your act of running is no-mind. Now, if you had to think about each letter you poke on the keyboard, your typing speed would slow dramatically, your conversation with your friend would suffer, and you would have no idea what the television program is about. And if you were to consciously think about the mechanics of every step as you jogged up the stairs, you would soon be face down and bleeding. Mushin occurs when you don't make a conscious effort to achieve it. Here is a simple exercise that gives you a feel for this thing that Bruce Lee referred to as "It."

Throw a tennis ball against a wall a few times, beginning with easy tosses and then harder and harder ones, so that it bounces back to you faster and faster. Now stop. If you did the exercise successfully, there was little or no thought process involved. You just tossed and caught, tossed and caught. Okay, do it again, but this time focus on drawing your arm back, moving it forward, releasing the ball, watching where it hits, watching how it bounces back, lifting your arm to catch it, opening your hand, and snatching it out of the air. Did you notice that it's a tad harder to catch the ball and that the overall process wasn't as smooth? Only by *not* focusing on all the steps, and just doing, will you once again perform smoothly and catch the ball more successfully.

As mentioned, Bruce Lee called Mushin, It. He said that if he got into a self-defense situation and seriously hurt his attacker, he would argue in court that he didn't do it, but It did it. Well, that is a nice plan, but unfortunately it would not hold up in court. The point Lee was making, however, was that his response would be so automatic, so guided by his subconscious, that his actions would be beyond his conscious mind. Mushin.

Mushin is a product of your training, hard conditioning drills that mentally engrain responses to various threats. To reiterate, if you try to force it, it won't happen. It happens when you don't try, when you just *do*.

Combat examples One of co-author Demeere's long-time private students regularly tries to surprise his teacher with a sneak attack. On one occasion, during the course of writing this book, Demeere was putting his sports bag in a locker when he heard a sound from behind him. Without looking, without thinking, without any conscious thought, Demeere snapped up his leg and effectively blocked his student's surprise kick.

"Much to learn, you have," Demeere said sagely to the student, in his best Master Yoda imitation. So, why did he use that specific block? He hasn't a clue. He does know that he didn't have time to think, turn and look. His leg just lifted and effectively blocked the kick as if it had a mind of its own, as if it wanted to protect him. That was Mushin and an example of how it works in a timing moment.

Christensen knows of a police officer who was walking his beat when he noticed a van parked in a No Parking zone. The officer stepped around the back corner of the vehicle intending to walk up on the driver's side and tell the man to move out of the zone. What the officer didn't know as he approached the window was that the driver, minutes earlier, had killed someone. The van door swung open, and the driver stepped out – holding a gun in his hand, raising it toward the officer. A fraction of a second later, a hole appeared in the driver's chest. Later, the officer said his first thought was that someone had shot the man for him, and he even looked over his shoulder to see who it was. It was then that the officer realized that he had his gun in his hand, and it was he who had reflexively, unconsciously, and with perfect timing, shot the gunman. A Mushin moment. A product of the officer's extensive training.

Competition examples Christensen used to travel to San Francisco to train with a kempo instructor and retired tournament champion. Actually, the man had retired twice, once in his 20s when a back injury prevented him from continuing to compete, though he was ranked number one at the time. Twenty years later, at 40 years of age, he decided it would be fun to try his skill on the new generation of fighters. Within months he was ranked number two above all the teens and 20-somethings. Then his old back injury flared up and he had to call it quits for good.

He was nicknamed Radar on the tournament circuit, aptly named since it seemed that he always knew where his opponent's opening would be. Whenever that hole appeared in his opponent's defense, Radar's backfist or inverted punch (a punch thrown palm-side up with the rear hand, usually to the opponent's ribs) would slam into the target with almost invisible speed. Radar said it didn't matter if his opponent exposed his head or his ribs, because he would hit whichever "as if by magic." If his opponent blocked, say, the backfist, then Radar would instantly hit the exposed rib cage. If his opponent blocked the rib punch, he would be rewarded with a backfist to the chops. Whenever an opening appeared - *Zap!* - Radar's fist was there. Mushin. No-mind. Radar said that he was often just as surprised as his opponent since he hadn't given the moment any conscious thought.

Radar's secret? Actually, there wasn't one. It was all a result of practice, lots and lots of hard practice, resulting in Mushin.

Realistic training   To respond without conscious thought when the heat is on, you must drill your basic attacks and defenses until they become part of you, just as breathing is part of you. When that window of opportunity opens... *ku-whack*! your technique is through it in the blink of an eye. But you must be wary of what you program into your subconscious. If you feed it faulty techniques - the wrong technique or poor body mechanics - it will spit out faulty techniques, just when you need them the most in competition or in a street fight. Ensure that your drill is the right response for whatever window of opportunity is given you.

For example, the classic karate block, while powerful, isn't fast enough to stop a boxer's jab. A slap-type block is far more efficient and much quicker. So, before you do thousands of repetitions of anything, make sure you are doing the right technique and doing it correctly in a training scenario that relates to competition or street self-defense. That is the only way to be sure that what you program into your mind will be exactly what the timing moment requires. Once you figure it out, train hard to make those techniques fast, strong and reflexive. Mushin.

Another way faulty techniques are engrained is when your training partner attacks without true intent. Typically, he throws a punch and leaves his arm extended so that you can do all kinds of fancy things to him, or he throws a kick that is so far away that it would never hit you. But a street thug won't pull his blows and he certainly won't hold one out there for you. Insist that your partner throw techniques right at you and close enough to hit you should you block poorly. Getting whacked is good feedback that you did something wrong.

Is there a downside?   Is it possible that training to ingrain could be counterproductive and even detrimental in your evolution as a martial artist? Might those responses be used against you? Yes.

Case in point: One of Demeere's top students had developed a powerful roundhouse kick and then trained to always respond with a spinning back kick when it got blocked. He had so drilled on this follow-up that it had become natural, automatic. Seeing that this might be a problem, Demeere sparred with him, continually baiting his student to throw his roundhouse kick so he could block it. Since Demeere had "read" his student's set pattern, he was able to easily block the follow-up spinning back kick, and then hit him quickly with a counter of his own. It wasn't that the spinning back kick was a wrong move, but it was that the student always used it when his first kick got blocked. After their sparring session, Demeere explained to the student what he saw him doing and they worked out a variety of other responses. Though his student understood his error, he had done such a good job programming his response into his subconscious that it took a while before he no longer automatically used that spinning kick.

While an automatic response is the first stage of Mushin, and is invaluable in a fighting situation, one lone technique might not be the best for every situation. Total Mushin is to be completely free in your mind. You still respond without conscious thought, but the technique isn't always the same, or at least it isn't executed the same way in every situation. The problem with training just one way, and always with basic responses, is that you won't develop the ability to unconsciously adapt to variations in a situation. To develop that unconscious ability, you need to explore a variety of ways to apply your techniques, such as changing the rhythm of application, the angles, executing them at high, medium and low levels, and applying them against different types of attacks.

Begin with subtle changes. When your opponent launches a technique at your face and then launches the same technique at your knee, look to see if that affects your response. Can you get by with a subtle adjustment of your response, or do you have to make a larger one? At what point do you have to switch to an entirely different one? While it's good to have one technique that works in a variety of situations, it's smart tactically to know when to adjust that one move and when to change to one that is more applicable.

Consider the lead-hand hook punch This is a classic boxer's technique, used in some karate styles, though it's so effective it should be incorporated in all of them. Let's look at a few timing moments using the hook. You are in a left-leg-forward fighting stance, as is your opponent. Situation A is a perfect lead-hook punch to the exposed target. Situation B, however, is similar, but just different enough so that the hook isn't applicable.

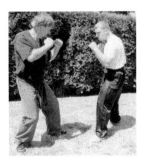 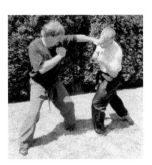

From an on-guard stance, launch a left hook into the cheekbone.

A. Your opponent drops his rear hand. Your lead hook immediately impacts the right side of his face.

B. Your opponent drops his left hand. Depending on the angle of his body and head, you might or might not be able to land a lead hook to his head. If not, your mind needs to be free to respond to the left side of his face with an appropriate technique.

A. You are leaning slightly forward as you clinch your opponent. He releases your arms and goes for a head grab. You immediately respond with a solid lead hook to his ribs.

B. You are leaning forward clinching and your opponent grabs you in a snug, arms pinned hold. Your mind needs to be free to respond to his open head area with a different technique.

A. You have tripped, slipped or been knocked down onto your knees. Your opponent steps forward to hit or grab you, and you seize the timing moment by hook punching the inside of his thigh.

B. You have tripped, slipped or been knocked down onto your knees. Your opponent steps forward but lifts his closest leg to deliver a finishing kick. Since you can't punch it, your mind needs to be free to respond with a different technique that best fits the situation.

While you have developed a fast and powerful lead hook punch, and you have thrown it a zillion times in basic drills, there will always be timing situations in which you can't use it; in fact, there will be lots of them. Your training must include as many variations as you can create with the hook, as well as situations where you have to abandon it quickly and use an entirely different technique. The skill and experience you gain from training in this fashion gives you the tools to *adapt* to the specific timing opportunities in competition and the street, as opposed to simply responding like a robot, and doing so ineffectively. In the end, when you train correctly, you increase the likelihood that you will respond to any window of opportunity, without conscious thought, with no-mind. Mushin.

A western approach to Mushin: Flow

In his book *Emotional Intelligence,* Daniel Goleman writes about a mental state he calls "Flow." He describes it as a condition where you are faced with a difficult challenge, physical, mental or both, that demands and requires total concentration, but is still within the reach of your skills and capabilities. You can be successful in the challenge, though it takes every ounce of skill you possess.

An interesting aspect of Flow is the balance needed between the pressure of the task and the attributes of the person performing the task. If it's too easy, Flow won't occur because there isn't enough pressure, and therefore no need for it. On the flip side, if it's too difficult, Flow won't happen if you lack the attributes needed to deal with the problem. Only when both the demands of the task and the capabilities of the performer are in a dynamic balance, will there be a chance of achieving Flow.

When you are in the Flow, you don't have to push your body hard to complete a task. Actually, you don't have to work hard at all. The Flow is often associated with a feeling of joy and pleasure; sometimes it's described as feeling like the task was too easy. "I feel great today!" fighters in the Flow often exclaim. Part of this feeling is derived from the balance between the workload and the effort applied to it, and part is due to total concentration on what needs to be done. There is no energy wasted on being afraid or worrying about whether it can be done, but rather all your mental and physical resources are used to face the challenge. You have confidence going into it because you know you are up to the task. The result is a kind of "knowing" that you are performing to the best of your abilities and that it's working out perfectly.

Flow in action   Demeere was sparring with a very tough opponent during a muay Thai class, and though he outweighed his classmate by at least 20 pounds, he couldn't match the man's speed and his ability to link techniques in ever-changing combinations. Whenever Demeere saw his opponent explode forward, he had only enough time to cover-up or side step the barrage of attacks that followed. But what Demeere lacked in speed, he made up in experience and precise timing. He would let his opponent land most of his attacks on his closed guard, his arms and fists, and wait for him to step back. As soon as he did, Demeere used the timing moment to attack with fast and short combinations, changing their rhythm each time to confuse and frustrate the other man. Though Demeere threw fewer techniques than his opponent, more of Demeere's landed.

Afterwards, onlookers said that they were surprised that neither of them had gotten seriously hurt since the intensity was so high. Demeere concurs that the sparring session was a hot one, but great fun, too. Both he and his opponent were willing to tear into each, and do so without malice. There was no conscious thought, just action. Blocks, counters and attacks flowed freely. Demeere recalls the moment as feeling great, because without any conscious effort, he had entered the Flow.

One time when Christensen was working patrol as a police officer, he received a radio call on an armed robbery, with a description of the suspect and the getaway car. Christensen was searching the side streets before going directly to the scene of the crime when he spotted the car blowing through stop signs. As Christensen pulled into a driveway to turn around, another police car roared by in pursuit. By the time Christensen caught up, the other officer had forced the suspect car over and was out of his car confronting the driver who had leaped out. As Christensen screeched to a stop, he saw the two scuffling, and the officer take a hard punch to his head knocking him back over the hood of his car.

A soon as Christensen scrambled out of his car, the suspect was on him swinging hard punches, all of which Christensen blocked as if they had carefully rehearsed the moment. When the other officer approached from the suspect's side, he again was punched and knocked back against the car. The suspect turned back toward Christensen, threw a kick, which was blocked and then another punch, also blocked. Christensen recalls only one conscious thought during the one-minute ordeal: "Enough is enough." He punched the man, breaking his cheekbone and exploding blood like a popped water balloon. The unconscious suspect fell to the ground.

Christensen recalls having no conscious thought as he blocked the man's kicks and punches. It was almost as if the fight had been choreographed, so smoothly did it go. Then when the one thought did pass across his mind – "Enough is enough" – he responded with an unplanned, perfectly executed and perfectly timed reverse punch. "I was in the Flow," he says. "It was almost fun. Well, okay, it *was* fun." The one flaw was that Christensen punched the man's head with a closed fist, something he has always taught students to never do. "Strangely, I didn't feel a thing; it didn't hurt my hand at all. I don't even recall the impact, though I do remember launching the blow. Like others have said: Being in the Flow felt great."

We said earlier that the surest way to lose Mushin is to stop and think about it. Well, the same is true with Flow. Should you stop and think consciously about what is going on, your mental resources will be drawn away from the goal and the all-important balance of workload and effort will be disturbed. It might not be by much, but it's enough to lose the Flow so that suddenly nothing works the way it should.

Our best advice is to just let it happen without forcing it. Train hard to be the best martial artist you can be and challenge yourself with ever more difficult exercises and tests. If you look for the right balance between the difficulty of the task and your skill at that exact moment, you will experience Flow. You don't have to be a black belt or great-grandmaster to experience it; even a beginner can do it. All it takes is finding the right challenge for your current skill level.

Now that you have a good understanding of the nuts and bolts of timing, the parts under the hood, the next stage is to examine the tools needed that make it work for you.

Seizing an opportunity

In essence, there are only two ways in which to apply timing: Either you create an opportunity or you take advantage of one. Applying this knowledge can be done in an infinite number of variations, as only your imagination and the depth of your knowledge and experience limit you. Though we distinguish two categories, there is a certain amount of overlap. It's best, therefore, to view these categories more as an integrated whole than as two separate entities.

Existing opportunities

Taking advantage of an existing opportunity is arguably the easier of the two methods. You don't have to do anything to make it happen because your adversary does all the work for you. However, you still have to recognize the opportunity when it appears. Since a timing moment is usually short lived, you have to be quick enough to act with the right response and do so before the moment disappears. The short duration of the opportunity and your quick and proper response are the main difficulties of taking advantage of your opponent. The solution to making this less difficult lies in your training. It takes time and lots of hard work to recognize all the possible opportunities that can present themselves in a fight. It's a skill that you will continue to improve upon for all the years of your martial arts training.

Knowledge increases options As a beginning martial artist confronting a front kick, you might think that a block and counter kick is the only response you can do. However, as you progress in your training, many other techniques become equally viable options to you: rushing the attacker as soon as you see the kick coming; moving off the line of attack and kicking his support leg; blocking his kick by stomp-kicking the attacking foot, and many others. What you never imagined yourself doing as a white belt can, months or even years later, turn into a favorite technique as you gain skill, confidence and experience. Remember how the backfist seemed weird when you first learned it, though now it's probably one of your favorite techniques?

Let's say you have never been good at the sidekick: you lack flexibility, your hips are naturally stiff, or your teacher taught you improperly. Whatever the reason, you rarely use the kick. Too bad, because one advantage of the sidekick is its effectiveness at long-range hitting. Properly executed, it can stop an advancing opponent in his tracks and keep him at a distance. Since you can't sidekick well, your sparring partners are constantly closing on you, and even scoring on you at a distance. It's one thing being scored on, but it's embarrassing to be scored on easily. It's even more humiliating when your opponents don't even bother protecting themselves since they know you can't reach them anyway.

Okay, enough with the blushing. You spend a month stretching hard and consistently, and working practical application drills with your once feeble sidekick. Thirty-one days later, it has turned into a usable weapon, so that now every time your opponents try to move in on you or try to hit you from a distance, your sidekick is right there saving the day for you. Great. But there is more.

The fact that you can now use that sidekick so well alters the way you view long-range fighting. The experience you gain with that one technique gives you valuable insight when using other long-range weapons, such as the front kick. As a result of your 31-day concentrated study, you now have a better sense of that range, which in turn can augment your understanding of medium, close and grappling ranges. Understand, however, that repetitive training isn't enough to attain this same knowledge. Merely mimicking a technique won't suffice. Now, don't misread this to think we are saying that repetitions aren't effective because they definitely are. But along with pounding out quality reps, you need to study, research and strive to comprehend what you are learning; strive to wring out every nuance of the technique, good and bad.

During Joe Lewis's reign of the tournament world, he was asked how he was able to score so often with his sidekick. His opponents knew he was going to use it, but still they got nailed with the kick virtually every time. His answer: "I never throw it the same way twice." Through constant training, Lewis had developed a total understanding of the sidekick, especially how to use it in a variety of ways. That should be your objective, too, so that in just a short while, your effort reaps extraordinary benefits.

Opportunities appear in many shapes and sizes, so you need the ability to first recognize them and then take all that you can from them. We suggest you experiment carefully with the following concepts:

- **What are the strong and weak points of your opponent's stance?** Is it a position from which he can easily explode toward you? Can he retreat quickly from your attacks? Will he need to first shift his weight? Is he covering potential targets well or does he leave them open? Is he leaving them open on purpose to trap you? What techniques are most available from his stance? When you can answer all of these questions and any others that you can think of, you are on the path to learning.

- **What are the strong and weak points of your opponent's footwork?** Observe your opponent's footwork to see how you can use it against him. Does he take steps that are too large? Too small? Is his body in balance as he moves, or does it lead his legs? Is his center of balance stable or does it move up and down, or sway excessively to one side or the other? Does he plant his weight heavily as he steps, which makes for stable but slow footwork, or does he dance excessively? Every error in your opponent's footwork can be a golden timing moment for you. Chances are he doesn't even know he makes errors, which will increase the element of surprise when you seize a window of opportunity.

- **Study your opponent to determine how well he controls his techniques**. A good fighter strikes like lightning and is gone before you know what happened, while a poor fighter inadvertently exposes opportunities for you to take advantage of during or after he attacks. Instead of putting his foot back on the floor after he kicks, does he posture with it in the air for a moment, or does he allow its momentum to carry him forward, more or less out of his control? Does he telegraph his attacks? Is his first technique in a combination sharp, while the ones that follow are slow, weak or sloppy? The more errors he shows in his techniques, the more windows of opportunity for you to attack.

- **Are his choices in techniques sound?** This is a rather broad question that encompasses many elements. Here are just a few. Does he consistently lead with hand attacks or with kicks? Does he mostly use lead or rear hand/leg attacks? Does he use the same ones, regardless of their effectiveness? Does he set them up with strategy or does he flail instinctively? Does he use the wrong technique for the range? The real purpose of your search for answers is to determine how you can make a perfect timing moment out of his errors.

- **How strong is his focus?** Some fighters start out strong but lack the mental and physical endurance to continue at the same intensity. Does he get mentally upset or frustrated when he misses? If so, where is the timing opportunity for you to exploit? Is he mentally zeroed in on you, or does he seem to fight on autopilot with little, if any, plan?

- **In a street confrontation, how easily is the adversary distracted?** Does a passing car make him look? Does he continuously look over to see if his buddies are enjoying his bullying moment? When you look to the side, do his eyes follow? These are all excellent timing moments for you to exploit.

- **Is the adversary cognizant of nearby obstacles?** Can you maneuver him in some fashion so that he trips over an unseen object? Can you charge him so that he backs up and trips over something? Can he be maneuvered in some way so that your buddies can restrain him? Learn to gather information quickly and then exploit a weak moment.

- **Is the adversary aware of nearby weapons?** Can you somehow maneuver him away from potential weapons? Can you position yourself so that you can grab an object to use in self-defense? Is there a chance his buddies will hand him a weapon, or that one of them will use one on you?

- **Is there an avenue of escape you can use?** Can you maneuver him away from the door? Always keep in mind that your best bet in a street fight is to avoid it by getting away from the scene. Swallow your pride and look for a way to grab the right moment to make a hasty escape.

Creating an opportunity

There is nothing terribly complicated about creating a timing opportunity, though we have seen some instructors come off as mystical and grandmaster-like on the subject. There is no need for that, but there is need for analytical observation and hard physical training. To create an opportunity, you simply manipulate your opponent into a specific position or manipulate him into reacting to something you do. Okay, it's not always simple, but it's never terribly difficult, either. For sure, there is nothing mystical about it. Once you get your opponent to do what you want him to do, the timing opportunity is right there for you. You might have to do something to him physically or you might have to play a trick on his thinking process. What you do and how you do it depends on the specific reaction you are trying to elicit. Know that it might work once but it's rare that an average to excellent fighter will fall for it twice. Here are a few examples.

- An assailant throws a right arcing punch at your head. You respond by stepping forward, while simultaneously covering your face with your left elbow and punching his shoulder with your right hand. You want to palm slap his groin but first you need to execute a transition impact. After punching his shoulder, your right fist draws back to begin the arc downward to his groin, smacking into the attacker's chin as it passes by. Without pausing or saying "sorry," continue the downward arc and execute a powerful groin shot. The clip to the chin fills the transition time with your blow rather than giving him an opportunity to hit you. It probably won't knock him out, but it will stun or distract him, providing you with a tad more time to deliver the big attack to his groin. *Practice 1 or 2 sets of 10 reps on both sides.*

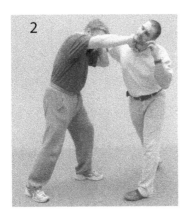

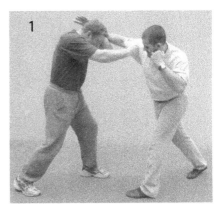

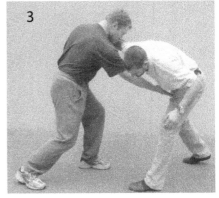

Block and counter punch the nerve in the front of his shoulder. Strike his chin as you whip your hand down and into his groin.

- One of the most feared weapons of the muay Thai fighter is his roundhouse kick to the thigh, commonly called "the leg kick." It generates its awesome power from a tremendous torque of the hips, fast footwork, and impacting with the hard surface of the shinbone. It's so powerful that a kicker can break his own shinbone when an opponent blocks it with a raised knee. To prevent this from happening, muay Thai fighters strive to use various approaches that manipulate their opponents into a position so they can't raise their legs to block. One way is to force the opponent to put his weight on the blocking leg.

For example, you and your opponent are both in left-leg forward fighting stances. To prevent your opponent from using his leg to block your killer roundhouse kick, you first throw a hard left hook punch to his head to make him momentarily shift his weight to his lead, left foot. To avoid losing balance, he either puts all his weight on his left leg or he takes a small step to the side. Either way, his balance is dependent on that left leg, and for a fraction of a second, he is unable to raise it or block with it. It's at that precise timing moment that your right-leg lands – and does so unblocked. In this case, you created a timing moment by manipulating your opponent into a position where he was unable to respond to your deadly leg kick. *Practice 1 or 2 sets of 10 reps on both sides.*

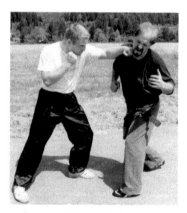
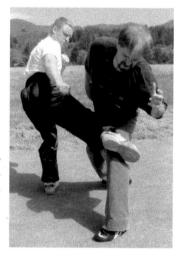

Slam a left hook into your opponent's face to make him shift his stance and weight to his left leg, to create an opportunity to whip a roundhouse shin kick across his thigh.

- Your attacker grabs you in a front bear hug and forces you backwards. Before he can fully lock his arms and squeeze, take another step backwards for stability as you simultaneously stab him in the groin with a spear hand. Most attackers reflexively pull their hips back, though there are some you might have to stab repeatedly or follow with the good ol' squeeze and twist. As he tries to pull away from the stabbing attack, his arms straighten, making his hold less powerful. To break free and daze him at the same time, lean sideways and snap your right elbow straight up into his chin. From there you can go into any number of strikes or grappling techniques, such as the arm lock pictured here. *Practice 1 or 2 sets of 10 reps on both sides*

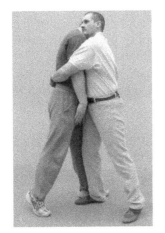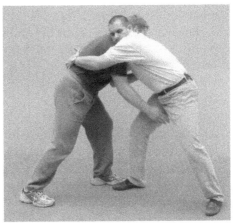

Your attacker grabs you in a front bear hug and forces you backwards. Spear him in the groin as you step back ...

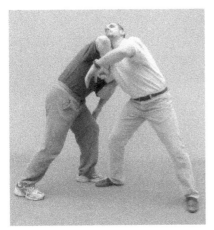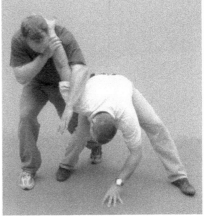

then take advantage of his weakened grip by popping him in the chin with your elbow. Finish with an arm lock.

All of these techniques show ways to manipulate your opponent's body and mind so you can take advantage of one or more windows that you have opened. Here are three categories from which to create your ideas and techniques:

- **Body manipulation.** The aforementioned lead-hook punch followed by a kick to the dominant support leg is a perfect example of forcing your opponent's body to go where you want it. By trick or physical force, you cause your opponent's entire body or just one of his limbs to move in a particular direction so that you can take advantage of the moment. The manipulation can be an offensive technique, such as the hook punch to the head, or it might be an intermediary action that sets up the timing moment you have in mind. It can be a two-count movement, such as a hook punch and round kick, or the timing opportunity might manifest itself after a combination of several moves. For example:

  o Hit him in the stomach to force his body to bend forward and then strike his exposed face.

  o Attack his eyes with a finger jab to force his head and upperbody to lean back, then punch or kick his exposed stomach.

  o Block your opponent's punch and then push his arm across his body to clear a path for a chokehold, either from his side or from behind.

  o Hook your opponent's lead foot or leg so that it widens his stance and exposes him to a groin kick.

- **Mind manipulation**. Here you force your opponent to think about something other than what you really want to do to him. This can be done with a physical move, with verbal tactics, or a combination of the two.

  o Point to a spot behind your aggressor and then attack when he looks or turns around.

  o In the middle of a sentence -- either yours or his -- attack his closest target. Because he was either listening or speaking, his reaction will be slowed ever so slightly as he begins a new OODA loop.

  o As he speaks, bring up your hand to your ear and lean forward, as you ask, "What?" When his mind shifts to repeat his words, use the close, ear cupping hand to strike his face.

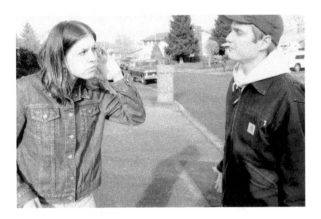

Lean forward slightly, cup your ear and say, "What?" as if you can't hear.

Then execute a brachial plexus stun against his neck with your forearm.

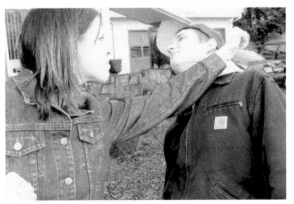

- **Feinting, faking and drawing.** This category combines the previous two by luring your opponent to react in a certain way that allows you to exploit him.

  - Feint an attack by snapping your head and torso slightly forward, but then return quickly to your original stance. Exploit your opponent based on how he reacts. He might have tried to counter attack and left himself open or perhaps he stepped awkwardly in an attempt to evade.

  - Fake a lead-hand punch to the face, and when he reacts with a raised block or even with a simple jerk of his head, follow with a rear-hand punch to his body.

  - Draw your opponent's fire by deliberately exposing an opening in your guard, such as lowering your lead-hand guard a little too much, leaving the front side of your face exposed. Be prepared to block or evade an attack there and then counter.

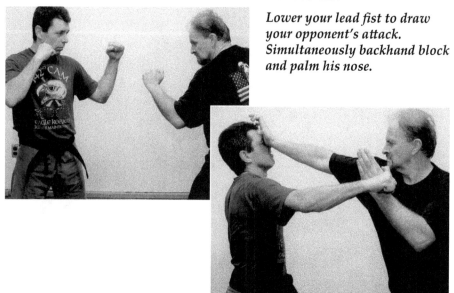

Lower your lead fist to draw your opponent's attack. Simultaneously backhand block and palm his nose.

Creating opportunities and taking advantage of existing ones are all about fighting smart. The opposite is to flail madly without a plan. Consider what karate and kickboxing champion Bill "Superfoot" Wallace wrote in the *Ultimate Kick*: "A lot of fighters use a technique I call 'throw and hope.' They'll take their stance and, using what their instructor said, throw a roundhouse kick. And it will probably be blocked. Now they're stumped. They have to think about what they'll throw next. They need to get away from that. Set up combinations, a master plan of plans within plans."

The ultimate goal of timing is to use the right technique(s) at the right time. Author and kickboxer Martina Sprague says, "Timing must be precise for optimum results. For example, an opening might exist for one or several seconds, but it is only during a precise moment that you will do the most damage. This involves the ability to be accurate with your strike or block." So, instead of attacking a target that is obviously closed to you, or attacking in such a way that your technique is almost always blocked, you are far better off looking for windows of opportunity or making those moments happen.

Choosing the right time

Let's look at "phases of timing," a useful tool in deciding when to seize a timing opportunity. There are three distinct phases during your opponent's attack in which you can react. Each one has its own characteristics with specific advantages and difficulties. Try to think of these phases as a sort of sliding scale as opposed to three absolute times in which you must act. There is lots of overlap between them and it's sometimes hard to see the difference. To help you visualize this concept, let's look at it on a timeline scale.

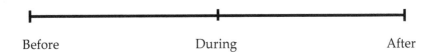

Before   During   After

The points on the line indicate the timing moment in each phase, though it's best to think of this as more of a teaching tool since it's often difficult to pinpoint the exact moment to act offensively.

After the attack is launched

Timing your response to land at the conclusion of your opponent's attack is used most often by beginning students. This isn't because it's easy, but because beginners don't have any other choice. They just don't have the training yet to react at another point. It occurs when you don't see your opponent's attack until it's near the end, or at the end, of the timeline scale. Success at this point is poor because your opponent has the advantage of having moved first. His attack accelerates in your direction while yours has yet to move, putting you in a position of having to play catch-up. Clearly this is difficult to do, especially if your opponent attacks with a clever plan, uses well-placed combinations, or does it on a day when you aren't at your best. For the average martial artist, or for a superior martial artist having an off day, timing a response after the attacker has committed his technique is difficult at best.

Actually, there are fighting systems that favor hitting at the end of the opponent's attack. Many of the internal martial arts (tai chi chuan and aikido, to name two) like to hit after the opponent attacks. They let the attacker commit to a specific technique and then use his technique against him. Their objective is to avoid having to use brute muscle power, and wait to exploit the attacker's energy after he has initiated his attack or he has been tricked into attacking. This requires skill and experience to predict or manipulate the opponent's attack and then seize the moment of opportunity.

Setting up a timing moment   Here are three tricks, if you will, to make this work for you.

- As you spar with your opponent, keep your guard up to protect your head. After a few minutes, pretend to tire and lower your lead hand to expose the side of your head. Stay alert and ready for your opponent's attack. There it is! A jab on a straight course for your nose. Instantly drop under his jab and counter with a technique of your choice.

- As you spar, deliberately stay outside of his kicking range as much as you can. Don't clinch with him and avoid all other close-range interaction and middle- range clashing. Your objective is to condition your opponent to you always moving away from him and always staying just outside of where he can kick you without having to close the gap. The average fighter will become frustrated and begin reaching with his kicks, causing him to lean a little when he sets down. As soon as you see this awkward and ever-so-brief moment, execute a fast sweep just as his kicking foot lands on the floor. And he will probably set it there, too, since you have conditioned him to think you won't engage at that range. Sweep and hit him.

- One of the most common attacks by the untrained fighter on the street is the ol' arcing haymaker, what co-author Christensen calls the John Wayne punch. It's a large, telegraphed punch that is about as subtle as an approaching train. Suppose you are at a party where a drunk is taunting you for some reason. You try to leave with your date, but the bozo follows you to your car. Because your gut instinct tells you not to turn your back, you face him and try using your verbal skills to end the confrontation. It doesn't work on his pickled brain, and suddenly he cocks back his right fist to wind-up a John Wayne punch that starts from waaaay back over his shoulder. Although you could easily rearrange his face, his big wind-up gives you enough time to decide to end the situation nonviolently and impress your date as to how you are a real humanitarian. You duck easily under the wide-swinging punch, shoot in for a takedown and apply a simple control hold.

Practice 1 to sets of 10 reps on both sides of all three scenarios.

During the attack

In this phase on the Timeline scale, you execute your technique *as* your opponent attacks, an effort that requires tremendous reaction speed. You can do it, though, because you have trained for it.

One of the primary advantages of hitting during your opponent's attack is that he is unable to respond. He launches a front kick toward your stomach and you, as quick as a wink, slap his leg off course and drill a backfist into his face. Or, even better, you angle off and hit so well that you don't even have to block his kick. Either way, it's hard for him to react to your action because there is a limit to how fast he can respond in the middle of his attack. He is committed to his kick, whether consciously or unconsciously and, as such, it's hard for him to change course physically and mentally to defend against your counter blow. Keep in mind that it's not impossible because a select few, elite fighters can do it.

To be clear, we are talking about your opponent's all-out, take-your-face-off blow, not his non-committed attacks, those designed mostly to test or bait you. The latter are typically found in sports fighting, where an opponent uses fast but powerless techniques, such as jabs and back-fists, to see how you react, or to lure you into exposing yourself to the nasty technique he has waiting in the wings. But street thugs use them, too, especially individuals who have had training, say in a community boxing program, or a few months of martial arts training. It's much harder for you to launch a counter during these "feeling out" attacks because they are usually fast and lack body commitment. The window of opportunity they present closes quickly.

The primary disadvantage of seizing a timing moment during your opponent's attack is the very real possibility of colliding with him. As difficult as it is for your attacker to change course when he sees your counter, it's equally difficult for you should you make a mistake in interpreting his action. For example, you see him chamber for a front kick and you angle off diagonally with a plan of punching him. It turns out that he chambers his roundhouse the same way, and now it's arcing on the same path you took to avoid his front kick. You try to change course, but it's too late. *Whump!*

Let's look at five situations in which you time your counter to land during his attack. The first three are relatively safe to do, while the second two carry an inherent risk.

1. As your opponent throws a right hook punch, you duck under it and deliver one of your own to his midsection.

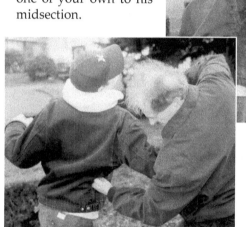

2. Your attacker swings wildly with his right fist. Duck underneath and close the gap at the same time, using your forward momentum to slam your forearm into his midsection and pull out his knees for a takedown.

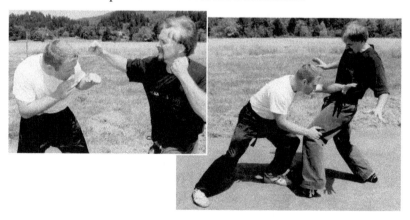

3. As he launches a roundhouse kick to your head, you angle off and sweep his support leg from under him.

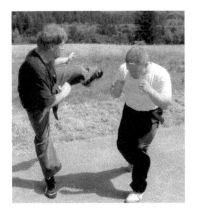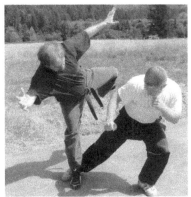

4. As he executes a reverse punch, you angle off and hit him with your jab.

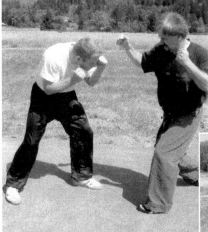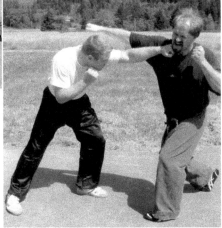

5. As he reverse punches your middle, you jab over and through his punch.

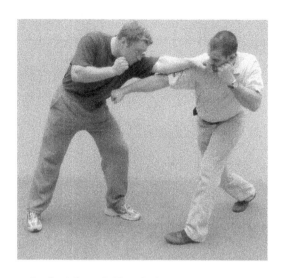

Practice 1 to 2 sets of 10 reps on both sides of all techniques.

In the first three examples, his attack and your well-timed counter don't cross, but follow parallel, though not converging lines, meaning there is no point where they intersect. This type of exchange, when countering during the opponent's attack, is the safest for you to do. By ducking and countering in example 1 and 2, you remove the target from the path of his punch, and in example 3, you are no longer in the path of his foot by virtue of moving your head as you shoot for a leg sweep. What is even more appealing is that his techniques leave him wide open for your counters, meaning there is less chance of you getting entangled or smothered by his moves since you don't cross paths. By the very nature of his attacks and the track of your well-timed counters, he is unable to protect himself. As stated before, it's difficult for him to switch gears from performing a full-power attack to first recognizing and then defending against your incoming counterattack.

Examples 4 and 5 illustrate crossing lines of attack: The lines intersect at a certain point and even "slice" each other. In example 4, you move the target off your opponent's attack line as you counter, but in example 5, you don't move offline or even block it, but rather go through his punch with your penetrating jab, albeit with a slight angle. Actually, you cut through the top of his forearm, using your forearm as you would a large knife. This forces his punch away from the target as yours heads for his face.

Crossing lines demands much better timing on your part and a solid understanding of the structure of your techniques. Obviously, you need a strong and stable technique to cut and divert his blow. If you lack the necessary timing skill or you use a technique to slice that is too weak for the task, you increase the chance of failing and getting whacked by your opponent's initial attack. When you time it right and choose a strong counter, it feels effortless. Your blow lands heavily as his just goes away. Try not to be smug.

It's called timing for a reason

Implementing perfect timing during your opponent's attack requires a keen understanding of the different lines and angles of attack on which techniques travel. Since selecting the exact moment to move and on which angle to move is so precise, running into your opponent's attack is a very real possibility. Knowledge of when to move and where to move comes from study and hard training. Most errors occur when you explode into action too soon, before you have fully identified the attack. This usually results in a collision. Conversely, when you take too long to recognize an attack, you gravitate toward the previous stage on the timeline: defending *after* he attacks.

Success is all about your skill, understanding, and the experience that comes from training specifically on timing your counter during the opponent's attack. You won't develop this ability by tomorrow. It takes time and training, but it's worth the effort because it feels so good to crunch your opponent at the very moment he expects his blow to land.

Before the attack

Hitting your opponent before his attack means that you must intervene at the earliest stages of the timeline. As mentioned earlier, it's sometimes hard to distinguish between the phases. If you see him set up to launch a backfist, and a half second later you attack, you are really countering in the middle of his attack. To attack him before, however, you must explode at the first indicator that he is about to move. Easy to say, but hard to do.

Of the three phases, this one is the most valuable from a practical point. If you flip back to where we discussed Boyd's cycle, you recall that action is generally superior to reaction. If it's you who is reacting, this means you are forced to go through the cycle as your attacker is completing his. In other words, you have the unfortunate task of trying to play catch-up and there is a real possibility you will fail. But by attacking before your opponent engages, you immediately increase the odds in your favor by sending him into a new OODA loop. In competition, you don't want to give your opponent the chance to score on you; so the quicker you hit him, the better for you. Yes, sometimes countering is a better strategy, but it can be more difficult to execute than striking first.

On the street, however, striking first gets a little sticky from a legal standpoint. Though you may be in the right, the legal system tends to frown on pre-emptive strikes, especially if you can't prove that you were going to be attacked. While striking first is a sound choice strategically, you should research your local laws before using this strategy on the street. So what do you do if it's illegal? You get real good at countering during or after your attacker's move.

Now there is always some guy in the back of the room who calls out, "I'd rather have 12 sit in judgment of me than have six pallbearers carry me." Nine times out of ten this heckler has never been dragged through the legal system. Trust us on this: It's nearly as bad as being carried by six pallbearers. Fortunately, in this case, you have a choice of two other options, or times, when you can hit. Therefore, polish all three.

A legal tip

Should you get into a real street confrontation, it's in your best interest to immediately write a "report" as to what occurred. Don't fabricate anything, even if you were not entirely in the right. Your report can be tossed out if it can be proven - by physical evidence and witness statements - that you are being untruthful, even if only in one or two sentences out of 50.

Articulate why you felt the attacker was about to assault you. Use your martial arts training to establish your reasoning. Write, "In my three years training in the discipline of karate, I have learned that when a person makes a verbal threat, clenches his fist, and pulls his shoulder back, he is about to launch a punch..." Detail everything the assailant said, including his facial expression, tone of voice, and body language. Note at what point he clenched his fist and drew his shoulder back.

Write in detail what you thought in that split second and why you decided to land the preemptive strike. Be sure to include that there was no avenue of escape or if there was, why you didn't think you had time to take it. Be accurate, be truthful and leave nothing out. Such a report can be a powerful document in your favor months later in court.

To strike an instant before your opponent attacks requires a mastery of range. It won't do for you to strike before he attacks if your poor choice of range allows him to easily counter you. You want to set up your counter so that your blow lands first, hard, and in such a way that he can't strike you back, or at least not until you are ready to block. Here are a few examples:

- Here is an old tournament trick, but a good one if performed intelligently. Even experienced fighters sometimes fall prey to it. After you and your opponent bow in for the match, assume your fighting stance and get mentally prepared to explode forward when the referee gives the signal to go. Although you are looking at your opponent, you are in tune to the referee's command. The instant he gives the signal to go, blitz into your opponent with the technique(s) of your choice. Be careful not to explode too soon; you don't want to get penalized. Move too late, however, and the surprise effect is gone. Ideally, you want to start moving at the referee's first utterance of his command. If it's "Go," start on the letter "g." Just be careful not to jump the gun, as it's easy to do.

  Many fighters are startled when you pull this trick on them, but in the event your opponent isn't intimidated, make sure your attacks are clean and quick, as opposed to barging in like an out-of-control rhino, leaving yourself open to counters. Be like a pouncing tiger: swift, efficient and straight to the objective.

  Here is what author and tournament champ Dan Anderson did when his opponent used this on him. "I fought this fellow I didn't know in Olympia, Washington, so I took him lightly. He hit me with the first points - *bang! bang!* - right on the referee's word, "Go." Going back to the starting line I knew he was going to charge me again. So, right as the official said, "Go," I fired a backfist. The next exchange I fired a rear hand punch. The last exchange I fired another back fist. He charged each time and ran into my strike each time. I knew that I had to throw my strikes right when the official said, "Go."

- Pick one or two spots on the mat or in the ring and make those places a visual cue on which you will respond with an attack. When your opponent moves over the cue and he isn't attacking, you attack him. This can be disconcerting to him because he doesn't know that you are going after him every time he is in a specific location, as opposed to going after him in response to something he is doing. Of course, you can't do it every time he passes over your designated spot, especially if he is attacking, or you are too far out of range. But if he isn't attacking and all conditions are good to go, hit him the instant he hits the spot. This works because you have created a cue to respond to, one that is mental and location oriented. This type of timing is most unconventional, which is why it works to surprise your opponent so well.

As you experiment with hitting after, during and before your opponent's attack, notice how they tie in with the aforementioned concepts of exploiting your opponent when he inadvertently presents a timing moment, and when you force him to make one for you. As you work with the various ideas and information throughout this book, the concepts of timeline and opportunities need to be kept in the forefront of your mind. Think of them as framework that supports everything else.

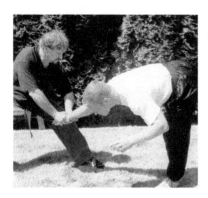

CHAPTER TWO

WINNING & SURVIVING TAKES PERFECT TIMING

The cramped space isn't desirable for either one of you, but it's worse for the person who is suddenly and abruptly attacked. Therefore, make him that person.

Good timing doesn't exist in a vacuum independent of all other factors. It needs other elements, gimmicks, tricks, and highly developed mental and physical attributes to make a timing moment more effective, more powerful, more explosive and, if the situation calls for it, more deadly. Let's examine several components to see how they can be combined with precise timing to ensure that the outcome of the fight is in your favor.

Fighting ranges

As martial artists we are far better off than the military when having to consider fighting ranges. At one end of the spectrum, the military trains at close range hand-to-hand fighting, and at the opposite end they train to fight at remote range with deadly laser beams emitted from satellites far above the Earth, all the while being responsible for every other fighting method in between these two extremes. In comparison, martial artists got it easy: We just have to train to fight with our body parts in kicking range, punching range and grappling range. (Sometimes you've to dig to see the bright side.)

The range diagram – circles of influence

By whatever name you call that bit of space between you and your opponent or adversary – range, distance, space or gap – knowing what to do and what not to do in it can mean the difference between winning or losing. Much has been written about distance in magazines, books and on internet sites, and for a good reason. Whether it's two martial artists clashing in the ring on Saturday afternoon or two high-tech fighter jets going at it over the sea, all fighting boils down to what takes place in that all-important space.

Most written data concerns *what* to do within the space but we are going to discuss *when* to do it. For our purposes, "when" means timing. If you think about it for a moment, fighting is all about "when," and "what" is almost secondary. It's often irrelevant whether you hit the guy with your foot or clobber him with a dead cat. What is relevant is when you hit him. If you miss-time your kick or your swing with that cat, the attack simply slices through the air, hitting nothing. Yes, you have a killer kick and yes, the dead cat would make an interesting splat against the guy's forehead, but since your timing was off, *what* you chose to attack with is irrelevant because you erred in choosing *when* to use the weapon.

Before we look at a few circles that help make the concept of ranges clear, let's make sure we are talking about the same thing when it comes to ranges. You can make more divisions than in this list, but generally these five suffice.

- **Out of range**: Neither you nor your opponent can touch each other.

- **Long range:** You can land attacks with techniques that travel a great distance, usually leg techniques, such as a sidekick and front kick.

- **Medium range:** You can use techniques that cover less distance from a place that is still a ways from your opponent. This is generally punching range.

- **Close range:** You can use techniques that require a short distance to travel, such as elbow strikes and head butts.

- **Grappling range:** Though sometimes lumped together with close range, grappling range is where you clinch and/or apply joint locks, leverage moves, and throws. It's still possible to use certain strikes at this range.

Using a range correctly means controlling the distance between you and your opponent and making sure that you use tools appropriate for the distance in which you find yourself. While the definitions of these ranges seem absolute, there is much overlap.

For example, elbows are generally considered close-range weapons. However, it's possible to use them in other ranges, too. In Filipino and Indonesian arts, it's common to use elbow attacks directed at limbs. This is often done at medium and long range against an outstretched arm, even when it's attacking you. It's important to note here that your opponent's limb moves into your elbow range, as opposed to you moving into close range to elbow him. Normally, you are already in close when an opportunity to elbow your opponent's head arises. In this case, your opponent's limb crosses that invisible line that defines close range. *Practice 1 to 2 sets of 10 reps on both sides.*

When your opponent launches a punch, you simultaneously check and strike it with the point of your elbow.

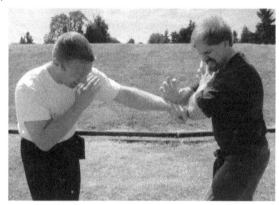

Some fighters like to catch a kick, a long-range-technique, and punish it with an elbow strike to the kneecap or thigh.

Block and catch your opponent's kick and drive your elbow into the vulnerable nerves just above his kneecap.

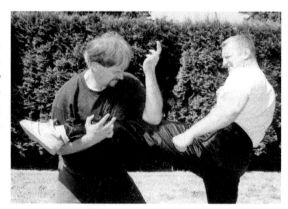

Christensen once had a student who liked to head butt and did so no matter where he was when the thought occurred to him. Even when he was outside of kicking range, he would charge his opponent as if possessed and butt him in the head. He even did jumping head butts, and more times than not, he made them work. As the old saying goes, rules are made to be broken. Know that with some exceptions, there are many techniques that can be used in ranges other than those in which they are normally used. This means that the definitions of the ranges aren't chiseled in stone. They are just another part of the puzzle that is fighting, and they should not be placed into too snug of a box.

Consider the following graphic.

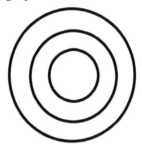

The concept behind this graphic is often called "Circles of influence," meaning that within each circle, you can influence what happens by using techniques best suited for that range.

The next time you train, imagine you are standing in the middle of this circle that represents the ranges, and take a few minutes to examine the reach potential of your various weapons. The inside circle represents close range, the second circle represents medium range, and the outer circle is long range. Go through all the ranges to determine the maximum reach with your techniques. Notice how some techniques can, to some lesser or greater degree, be applicable in different circles. For example, the largest circle, long range, is where you are most effective with your front or sidekick. The smallest circle is where you most effectively use grappling techniques, head butts, knees and elbow strikes. Once you move beyond that circle, other tools are better for the job. For example, a head butt works best in the closest circle but is less effective in the outer circle (Christensen's student the rare exception).

So far we have only examined your circle of influence, your range possibilities. It gets interesting when you combine your circle and your opponent's circle. There are only two possibilities when you and your opponent are in the same room: Either the circles touch or they don't.

Look at these graphs:

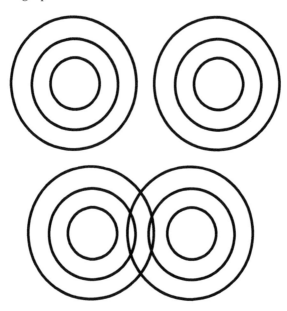

The first graph depicts both opponents squared off at each other, but out of reach. Their circles of influence don't touch and therefore they can't effectively attack each other, at least not without telegraphing their intention. Fighting at a distance is a common tactic for those who have great speed since they have the ability to zip in and out of striking range, doing damage and not getting hit. Should you face a fast opponent who stays at a distance, you need to read his intent so you are able to apply good offensive or defensive timing. Know first that in addition to his speed, he needs excellent footwork to close that space and zap you, and then get back out before you can react and hit him. Your success depends on your ability to anticipate his charging attacks and time your response. Arguably the best way is for you to let him commit to his attack and then either move in or angle away from him, as you counter. For sure, you don't want to let him commit while you just stand there because he is too fast for that, and never ever do you want to play the other fighter's game.

In the second graph, both fighters have moved closer so there is some overlap of the circles. It's in this area that both opponents can influence each other, meaning they are at the right distance to land attacks. The closer they come together, as the area of overlap becomes greater, the more ranges become available. At first, only the long-range circles overlap, but as you move ever closer, medium and close range circles overlap. The more both circles of influence touch each other, the more techniques there are available. If the circles are completely overlapped, that means you are busy grappling.

Understanding range means you have developed a working knowledge of when your circles of influence overlap and you know the best weapon for the moment of opportunity. Know that overlap is never static. As you and your opponent move about, moving towards each other and moving away from each other, the overlap continually changes.

As noted before, executing an elbow at kicking range just might be the last technique you try, since a smart opponent will clobber you for your poorly thought out effort. Likewise, you can't throw a sidekick when clinching, as there is not enough room to chamber and launch. Try, and your opponent will whack you again, probably as he laughs. Precision timing is to know when to attack and what technique to use depending on all the existing elements, especially range. Think: *the right technique at the right time.* The trick, the skill, and the art is to progress safely from one range to the other. Understanding timing helps you do so successfully, without eating your opponent's foot. Lets look at two examples:

• You are out of range and rush in to shoot an elbow to the face. He sees your charge and your intent, and he easily kicks you in the groin.

• You are out of range and step in quickly with a feint to the groin. He reacts by leaning forward and covering his midsection. You quickly take another step and plant an elbow strike into his face.

The first example shows a poor understanding of range. Trying to set up a close range technique from way outside is a disaster waiting to happen. Because you rushed your opponent without first setting him up, you had to streak across long and medium ranges before entering close range where your elbow strike is most applicable. Passing through these outer ranges without doing something to keep your opponent busy gives him plenty of time to formulate a plan and put it into action.

In the second example, your goal is to deliver that same elbow, but this time you pass through the ranges actively. You step into range with a fake to his groin, which draws your opponent's attention away from his head as he leans forward to block. But his leaning action actually moves his head, your intended target, a little closer, so that you only have to scoot in a little to elbow him in the snout.

Say your opponent crosses the ranges to get you. He might use a long-range attack, a kick that you block so hard he loses his balance and falls forward into close range. You can't hit him at medium range because you are busy blocking his kick, and his loss of balance prevents him from attacking you, anyway. It all works out in your favor when he stumbles into close range, and you say poetically, "Hell-o. Eat my el-bow."

Know your reach capability

Unless you have poor vision or some other debilitating problem, you possess a built in distance detector that allows you to reach for objects and walk from point A to point B with accuracy. Without having to think and calculate, you can reach over and take hold of your cup of coffee. Without thought and without having to confer with a calculator, you can guide your body around a table without banging into it and knocking off the lamp. When you were a toddler, however, your distance detector had yet to develop, so you probably ran into the table as you staggered across the floor and you overextended when you reached for your glass of milk and knocked it over. But through physical and mental maturity, and experience, you grew out of that awkward stage so that now you function with a certain amount of grace.

The ingraining of distance perception for normal day-to-day activity, combined with your perception of distance developed through your martial arts training, has provided you with an excellent read of how close you have to be to punch or kick your opponent. You have also developed a highly tuned sense of your opponent's reach capability with his weapons, just as he has of your reach potential. So, since you both have a basic knowledge of each other's reach, which is a little like saying, "When all things are equal," to be the victor you need to do something contradictory to what he knows.

Modifying your reach

Although there are many ways to make yourself superior to your opponent, one way is to analyze your bread-and-butter techniques, the ones you use the most often, to see how you can modify some or all of them to get greater reach. With more reach capability, especially greater than what your opponent thinks you can do, the more windows of opportunity become open to hit. For example, many times your opponent drops his guard and glances away because he thinks he is out of range, so you don't attempt to hit him because you think the same. Well, you don't want to do anything to change his thinking, but you definitely want to change yours, which you do by "lengthening" some of your offensive techniques. Here are three ways to get an additional four to 24 inches of reach out of three basic techniques.

Reverse punch   This is a basic punch found in most systems, though many styles, by virtue of the way they execute it, limit its power and reach potential. Let's examine a simple twist on this old technique, one that more and more fighters are discovering provides greater extension and impact.

Assume a left-leg forward fighting stance and launch your right fist. For now, don't step forward with your lead leg so that you can get a clear picture of the technique's reach. Many traditional styles rotate the upper body until the shoulders are square to the front, a position that is limiting. Here is a way to go beyond this point, while remaining in balance and still able to flow into other techniques.

- Continue to rotate past square until your chest is facing almost all the way to the left.

- As your fist nears full extension (actually, just short of full extension since you should never lock your elbow), lean your upper body 10 to 15 degrees forward...

- ...and sink your lead knee two to four inches.

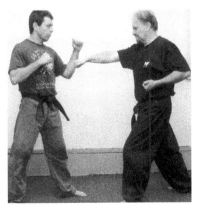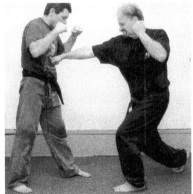

The body twist and knee sink adds, depending on your height and arm reach, six to 18 inches over the so-called classic, shoulders-square-to-the-front, method. This is an incredibly powerful punch and the beauty of it is that there is no sacrifice of stability; your balance is still intact. With just this slight modification, you get greater impact and greater reach, enabling you take advantage of timing opportunities that you would have otherwise missed.

The I-don't-want-to-fight pose   Here is a practical, yet unassuming fighting stance (sometimes called the "deescalation stance") that works great in the street. Stand with your body at a 45-degree angle to the threat with your hands up and open. "Let's talk about this," you say to the agitated person. "There is no need for violence." But he continues to badger with threats to do you physical harm. "I don't want to fight," you say, leaning back a little, your hands resting on your chest.

While your opponent basks in what he thinks is his intimidation of you, in actuality you have positioned yourself to blast him from a range that appears to be too far away. But look at the photos. Though your upper body leans back and your hands are drawn in close, your feet are still close enough to put you in easy striking range. When an opening appears -- a timing moment that you want to seize -- you can kick with your closest foot or you can roll your upper body forward as pictured, and gouge his blue eyes.

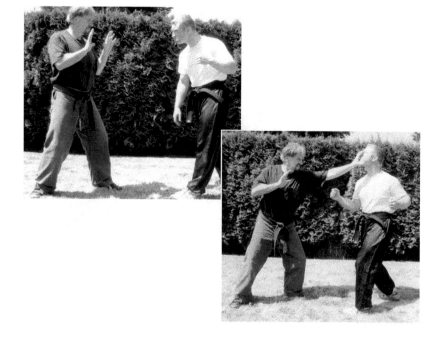

Slap kick As the name describes, this lead-leg kick is executed in a slapping motion, impacting with the top of the foot against the opponent's groin, or his face, should he be bent over. Assume your fighting stance with just a little more weight on your rear foot, but don't make it obvious. You don't need to chamber your lead leg to kick because it's already bent and itching to go. To set it off, simply lift your knee slightly and snap your lower leg up so that the top of your foot (the shoestrings area when wearing shoes) impacts the target. Striking with your lower shinbone hurts, too.

To gain an additional 12 to 18 inches of reach without taking a telegraphing step, sink your support knee two to four inches, simultaneously rock your pelvis forward, lean your upper body back a little, and snap your kick toward the target. With a little practice, you can pop this kick with good speed and balance while surprising the heck out of your opponent who was convinced you were too far away.

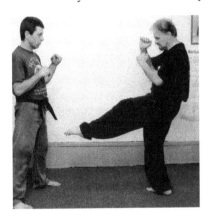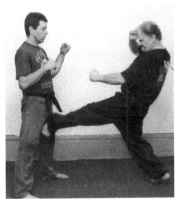

These are three examples of modifying your range done with two offensive techniques and a stance. If you have a few favorite techniques, analyze them as to how they can be tweaked to fool your opponent into thinking you are farther away than you are. Do a good enough job and he will relax his guard, thinking he is safe as he presents a window of opportunity for you to clobber.

Don't "overpull" your blows

Speaking of ranges, if you regularly pull your kicks and punches two to four inches from your opponent during practice, know that you aren't doing yourself any favors. Some schools practice in this manner out of tradition and some do so because of a ruling by their insurance company (typical of martial arts classes taught in health clubs). Traditions can be changed, but insurance company rules are based on the reality that we live in a litigation driven society.

Know that how you train is usually how you will fight in reality when your adrenaline is boiling and your heart is thumping. If you have trained to "over miss," and you never work on the heavy bag or hand-helds, or you never practice hitting a well-padded opponent, there is a good chance you will pull your blows under stress. Anecdotal evidence has supported this for years.

If training more realistically isn't an option at your school, and it's the only school you can go to, consider meeting with one or two fellow students away from class on off days and train with light to medium contact.

Let's look at a drill in each of the four ranges – kicking, punching, elbow and knee, and grappling – that helps you to not only see an opening and timing opportunity, but respond to it. Feel free to draw on your creativity to come up with even more.

Kicking range

There are actually two ranges in which you can kick. The first is where you are close enough to hit the target without stepping; the second range is where you can hit only after closing the distance with a step. Kicking without taking a step is usually faster though weaker than kicking with one. Let's look at a simple drill you can do with and without stepping.

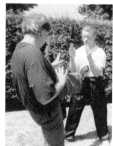

Which kick drill?   Stand before your partner in your fighting stance and close your eyes. Your partner's task is to choose one of four hand positions that indicate which kick to launch at him. For the sidekick, he holds both arms horizontal, one over the other a few inches apart. For the front kick, he holds both

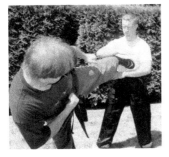

arms vertically in front of him, a few inches apart. For the roundhouse, he holds either arm along his side. For a groin slap kick, he extends his bent arm at groin height, palm open and facing downward.

When your partner makes a noise, such as clicking his tongue or snapping his fingers, open your eyes and quickly execute whatever kick is indicated by his arm position. At first, your partner presents the target for three seconds. As you improve, he presents it for only two seconds, then one second. If you don't get the kick in, your partner dissolves the pose and steps back (and laughs at you).

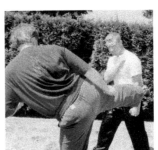

Practice 3, 2-minute rounds, alternating places with your partner.

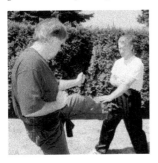

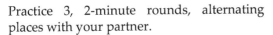

Punching range

As with kicking range, there are also two distances in which you can punch: one where you can deliver a hand technique without having to take a step to close the distance, and one where you have to lunge across a gap to hit. Let's look at a fun drill in which you respond with the best technique for the timing moment, stepping when needed or not stepping when you are close enough.

Statue This drill works best with three people: two to do the exercise and one to call out commands; let's call this person the sergeant. Though the drill can be practiced with kicks, let's simplify it for our purposes here and just make it a punching drill.

Begin by deciding who is designated A and who is B. The sergeant barks the command, "Fight!" that sets you and your training partner sparring at your choice of slow, medium or fast speed. On the sergeant's whim, he calls out "Statue!" which commands you and your partner to immediately freeze in place, no matter how awkward or silly looking your pose. You might be in mid punch as your partner is leaping to the side, with one of his arms up and one down. That is okay because the objective is to freeze instantly. Then, the sergeant calls out either A or B. "A!" he yells, which commands A to punch B, without hesitation, into whatever opening B has exposed given his frozen position. The sergeant then calls "Fight!" which commands you to resume sparring. The drill continues with the sergeant calling "Statue," then whichever letter he chooses, and then "Fight!" Continue for as long as you desire.

Practice 2 to 3, 2-minute rounds.

Statue improves your timing in two ways: It helps you to first recognize a target and then to hit it with the best weapon for the moment. Some examples:

• His lead hand is just below his chin and his head is leaning close to your frozen lead hand. Hit him with your lead.

• His rear hand is at his solar plexus and his lead hand is next to his ear, exposing the side of his head. Hit him there with a hook punch.

• His arms are positioned so that there is a four-inch gap between them, exposing his solar plexus. Drive home a reverse punch.

Secondly, the drill improves your ability to instantly hit an exposed target. At first, the target partner stays frozen for a three count: one thousand one, one thousand two, one thousand three, a time span in which the fighter has to hit the exposed target. After you and your partner have practiced the drill for a while and have developed a good ability to nail a target within the time limit, reduce the exposure time to two seconds. When the two of you can do that well, drop the time to one second. Then a half second. If at any time the hitter doesn't hit within the time given for the exposure, too bad, because the sergeant calls "Fight!" and the hitter is shamed forever for having missed the opportunity.

If you have been having trouble with target recognition, you will enjoy incredible improvement after just two or three training sessions with the Statue exercise. *Practice for a minimum of 10 minutes.*

Elbow and knee range

Although we call this range "Elbow and knee," it's also head butting, hip thrusting and shoulder ramming range. As in most timing situations, a door suddenly opens revealing a path to the target. When it happens at this range, however, your weapons are already virtually on top of the target.

Hit when the path appears You and your partner assume a clinching position. The drill is for you to take the path of opportunity when presented by your partner. Begin by jostling around as you normally do in a clinch. Your partner should deliberately lift an arm, lower it, or move it across his body as if to grab you in some fashion. The instant you see the exposed path to the target, execute an elbow strike (it helps if you know a variety of angles).

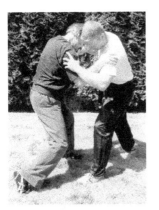 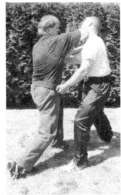

You and your partner clinch. When you detect a weakness in his hold, fire in an elbow.

You also want to monitor your clinch for an opportunity to deliver a knee strike, which is a tad harder than hitting with your elbow since one leg in the air requires solid balance. Recognizing a timing opportunity is a combination of seeing it and feeling it, meaning you know you can execute it given your balance at the particular moment.

Practice the drill for 2, 3-minute rounds.

Grappling range

Most often, fighters think of the grappling range as a place that is close and tight, snuggling close, if you will. This is true, but grappling range can occur at a greater distance, too. When an overly drunk person throws a huge, arcing haymaker punch that misses you by a foot, and it throws him off balance, that can be a grappling moment, though he is at middle or long range. Yes, it's a punching and kicking moment, too, but should you want to grapple with him because his arm is extended toward you and just begging to be grabbed, it's an option. Here is an example of a long-range grappling technique you can practice.

Timing an overreach   Assume an I-don't-want-to fight stance, hands up with your body relaxed as you face your opponent who is standing a little more than arm's reach from you. When he suddenly reaches, as if to grab you by your shirtfront, take a quick step back so that he grabs only air. Let's freeze-frame that for a moment.

Notice how his body leans forward slightly (if it's a good day, it's leaning a lot forward) and that his hand is right there for you to grab. Your balance is perfect and your desire to dump him is high. It's a perfect timing moment. Okay, remove freeze-frame. Grab his wrist. If he is very off balance, you can probably execute the move with just your one hand, but if he is slightly overextended, you would be wise to grab him with two. Jerk his arm down at a 45-degree angle between his feet and try not to smirk as his body splats onto the floor. *Practice 1 or 2 sets of 10 reps on both sides.*

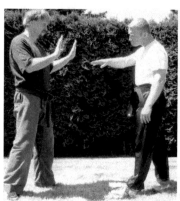 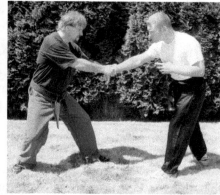

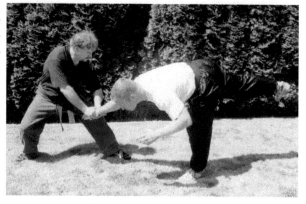

Your opponent is jabbing his finger at you. When it appears he is reaching for you, step back so that he over reaches a little. Grab his wrist and yank his arm down to the front in the direction of where a third support leg would be.

There are many other grappling techniques you can do at this remote range, such as finger lock takedowns, elbow drag takedowns, and wrist flex takedowns. Our point here is to just remind you that grappling range doesn't always mean up close. Now let's look at a training idea when you are close enough to hug your opponent.

Learn to read his point of unbalance You two are clinching again. Now, there are all kinds of ways to clinch, from the very formal judo style to two fighters clinging desperately to each other as they slam into garbage cans in an alley. The beauty of this exercise is that it doesn't matter how you grab as long as you can feel his weight distribution. So grab each other and commence dancing about (music optional).

Neither of you are trying to take the other down, but rather using the time to experience the other's balance at any given moment. Your partner's task is to move about and even exaggerate at first as he bends a little this way, leans into you, and then pulls back some. Your task is to learn to perceive each of these moments. Feel them happen. Read them. Allow a response to flitter across your mind, but don't actually execute it.

After you have practiced a few times with your eyes open, try it with them closed. Now, you have to rely only on your sense of touch, of feel. He dips a little to the right, feel that. He shifts his weight into you, feel it. After a few minutes, allow a response to flitter across your mind. He leans into you, imagine your hip slamming into his lower belly and flipping him over your shoulder. He leans to your left, imagine checking his right foot with your left and pulling him the rest of the way over. Here is an easy technique Christensen used often as a police officer.

Assume a clinch with your partner. As you jostle about, one of your hands is either behind his neck or gripping a wad of shirt or jacket collar, with your other on his upper arm. The instant his weight shifts forward and into you, jerk both your elbows in a straight line toward the floor. Do this quickly and sharply. Think of your energy as laser beams shooting out from your elbows and into the floor. Oh yes, step back a little to allow him to fall without banging heads with you. *Practice 1 or 2 sets of 10 reps.*

If you are thinking of other techniques you can do in the four ranges we discussed -- great. Our objective here is to remind you of the ranges and get you thinking of what all you can do in them.

Positioning

Thus far we have been talking about getting into range so you can seize an opportunity to zap your opponent. Being in striking range is one thing but getting there safely and into a strategically sound position where you can hit without getting hit is quite another. Even if you get into range without getting bonked, that doesn't automatically mean you can score a blow, as he might move quickly into a position of strength where he has the advantage. He can do this by outmaneuvering you or smothering your movements just before he hits you. At that moment, he has "frozen" your circle of influence. You are close enough to hit him, but incapable of doing so without first freeing yourself from his paralyzing influence. Consider these situations:

- Your opponent closes on you, jams your arms and jostles you about to keep you off balance. Though you are within range to hit him, he controls you so you can't.

- You are in a clinch with an attacker. Just as you get ready to hit him, he applies an elbow lock on your punching arm.

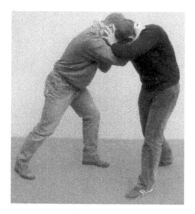 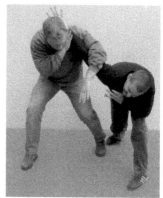

While clinching your opponent starts to punch,
but you quickly apply an elbow lock on his arm.

These examples show that being in range isn't enough. If you find yourself "frozen on the spot," that is, you are within range but you can't do anything, you either timed your attack poorly, you didn't time your counter well, or your opponent did a good job outmaneuvering you. However it happened, your opponent is one happy camper.

To avoid having a happy camper for an opponent, strive to position your body at the right distance and at the best angle to him.

The right distance

If you are too close or too far away, your techniques will either fail or you will have to change your game plan, which circumstances might or might not let you do. The next time you watch a boxing match, or any other full contact match, notice how many techniques fail or have little effect because they were fired from a position too close or too far away. Punches miss by several inches and kicks get smothered. Some of this is bound to happen in the heat of competition or in a knock down drag out in the street. But by training with position awareness, and being cognizant of positioning when the fight is on, you greatly increase your chance of being successful.

The best angle

Angle refers to the orientation you have in relation to your opponent. Consider these variations.

- You are facing him or standing sideways to him.

- He is either sideways to you or facing you.

- You both have the same feet forward or are in opposite stances.

- You are standing directly in front of him or you are at a 45-degree angle to him.

The angle at which you are positioned in relation to your opponent determines whether that position is weak or strong. A bad position is when your opponent is behind you pounding happily on the back of your skull. A strong position is when you are in front of him, attacking him with minimum force, while achieving maximum effect. Here are more examples:

- Lean your body away to avoid your opponent's high kick and then step in as his leg passes by. His force and hip rotation turns him sideways to you, or if it's a good day, he spins all the way around, exposing his back. Take advantage of his awkward, possibly helpless, position and dump your full arsenal on him.

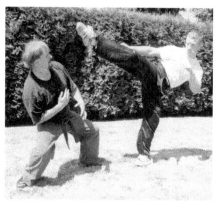 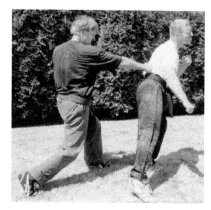

- Say the attacker throws a right cross. Slip to your left as you raise your right arm as a shield. Then move towards him from that side, pressing your right arm with your bodyweight against his right attacking arm, forcing it against his upper body. Your objective is to push it across his left arm so they are crossed. Keep enough pressure on him so he is forced to lean or step back. He is now yours to make him wish he had never been born.

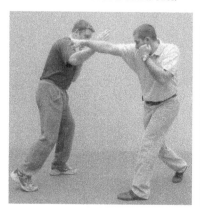 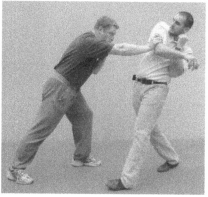

Practice 1 or 2 sets of 10 reps on both sides.

The particular angle you and your attacker find yourselves in at any given moment determines the offensive and defensive possibilities. Even the choicest angle won't win the fight for you, but it's a window of opportunity for you to jump through as quickly as you can. Choose the best technique for the job and you dramatically increase the odds of defeating your opponent.

Superior positioning also decreases your need to rely on speed, which is helpful if you are cursed with lots of slow-twitch muscles.

When you constantly maneuver yourself to the most advantageous angle, your opponent is unable to plot against you since he is kept busy thinking defensively inside his OODA loop. Say he is a circler, always moving to his left. For a moment, you pretend to let him control the motion by also moving to your left. Then you stop suddenly and move quickly counterclockwise to your right, directly into his path and attack. If he is slow to respond or he doesn't respond at all, the situation is what we call, "a walk in the park": Easy and pleasant for you. By not playing his game of moving about aimlessly, but instead thinking about positioning, you control the fight, and ultimately the outcome.

Many fighters, even experienced ones, have a tendency to go toe to toe and slug it out, similar to two mountain goats banging and locking horns, a style that rarely allows for clever positioning and opportune timing moments. In this crude approach, it's usually the fighter who has the most strength, endurance and willpower who determines the outcome of the fight. It's far more effective to think in terms of strategic positioning, fighting as if you were playing chess and thinking several steps ahead and working to continuously put your opponent in OODA loop after OODA loop. It's a smarter way to fight in competition and in the street, and lots more fun when sparring a classmate.

Framing with footwork

When framing, you actively control your opponent to create timing opportunities for you while reducing his timing opportunities. It also helps you determine when and where to move, something too many fighters do too randomly. The concept of framing is used often in ring competition and, with a few minor adjustments, can be applied to the street. The small set of rectangles on the left represents your feet and the set on the right represents your opponent's.

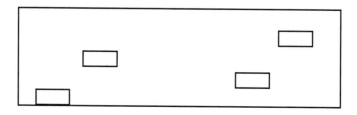

You are both in your fighting stance, just outside of kicking range. Your task is to visualize a rectangular frame around the two of you, as shown in the diagram, and imagine that it's attached to you, and only you. When you move, it moves, and when you stand still, so does the frame. No matter which direction you and your opponent step, you must mentally adjust the distance and positioning to keep him inside your imagined frame. If there is, say, four feet between you and he advances by one foot (remember, the frame doesn't move when he does), you must retreat one foot to maintain the frame.

This requires continuous monitoring and sound footwork to keep the distance between you constant. This isn't terribly difficult, but it gets tricky when trying to maintain the correct angle. For example, should your opponent start to circle to your left, taking a simple step forward to follow him won't be enough, as you must also turn a little to continue facing him. How much you turn and step depends on his action. If he circles quickly, you might have to make your movements fast and big, and vice versa should he make his circle small.

So far in this scenario, all you have done is maintain the same distance between you and your opponent, using the concept of framing to position yourself outside of his reach. You can't do this forever. Sooner or later you have to get down to beating your opponent with kicks and punches, meaning you have to start thinking and acting offensively. Once again, we start with adjusting the distance.

The easiest way is to simply move forward until you are in range for your kick or punch. As you advance, the imagined frame moves with you. If the other fighter doesn't move, the frame looks like this.

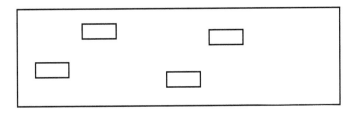

You have closed in and you are ready to blast him...then he moves. If he moves toward you, he will be in range faster than you expected. This is always a possibility in fighting, so it's critical that you be mentally prepared and ready to act. Let's say he took that forward step not knowing you were stepping forward, too. This surprises him and he immediately steps backwards to get away from you. No problem, you just take another step forward and clobber him. Be careful so as not to run into a counter technique.

It gets more problematic should he move to the side, though you can get tricky and "cut the corner." Your opponent is at 12 o'clock and you are at 6. He suddenly circles to his left toward 3 o'clock. Instead of just following him by moving to your right to 3 o'clock, you intercept him by streaking toward 2 so fast he is unable to stop and move away from you. By moving to 2, you don't have to adjust your position much more than if you were to go towards 3, and it's easier to keep him within your frame. Though he thinks he is moving a safe distance from you, keep him within the frame and surprise him with a hard charge *before* he reaches his destination. Now, don't just charge to 2 o'clock and smile at him, but lead the charge with a barrage of techniques. By cutting the corner, you open a window of opportunity, a perfect timing moment to blast through and land some thumpers. This takes practice, especially footwork.

Centerline

Centerline is a concept used often in Chinese and South-East Asian martial arts. So that we are on the same page, here is our definition of it: The centerline runs vertically through the center of your body, dividing it evenly in half from the top of your head, down through your torso, between your legs, and straight into the ground.

The concept can be used for a number of functions in the fighting arts, all of which relate to timing. Let's talk about centerline as it relates to controlling our opponent's attacks, his body, and to further our understanding of executing a takedown technique.

To control the opponent's attacks

Your timing improves when you force your opponent to attack to either the left or right of your centerline. As we explained in Chapter One, the fewer possibilities you have to monitor, the faster you can react.

To give yourself more time

By using centerline to control his body, you buy more time to do whatever you want to do. If you can't immediately score on an opponent or immediately debilitate an assailant on the street, being able to control his body via centerline gives you a little more time to set up a timing moment.

Make grappling easier

Your grappling techniques become more effective when using the concept of centerline because they are easier to do and take less time to apply

Here are just a few ways to make centerline work for you in a timing moment.

Order from chaos

Fights tend to be unpredictable and chaotic with fists and feet flying all about, often making it impossible to see the big picture. One of the most difficult aspects of fighting is to determine which attack your opponent is going to use: A right hook? A left roundhouse kick? The possibilities are many and it's impossible, no matter how experienced you are, to recognize each individual attack in a fraction of a second. Therefore, a system is desperately needed to simplify things, to make the burden of defending your life a tad easier. The centerline concept goes a long way toward giving us just that.

The centerline concept made easy Assume your fighting stance with your arms positioned on centerline, and hold them there as your opponent prepares to attack.

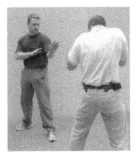

For him to hit you, his technique must come from either the left or the right. Pretty simple. Now let's toss into the mix another concept: The shortest distance between two points is a straight line. This concept combined with centerline gives you an advantage. As you control your centerline, your opponent is forced to go around your arms using circular moves that take extra time to get to you, such as hook punches and round kicks.

By controlling your centerline, you force the attacker to take the long way to get to you, while you enjoy countering using the shortest route to get to him. Since you only have to move straight forward, it appears that you are faster than your opponent, even if you aren't (we won't tell him if you don't.) This makes for a huge advantage when timing your counter, one that is likely to decide the outcome of the match or a real fight in your favor. Sounds simple in theory but to do it well takes practice, a lot of practice. Try this drill to get a feel for what this means.

Centerline drill Assume your on-guard position and place both hands on your centerline, using whatever hand placement you like -- palms up or down, hands low or high, but in this instance not too high or low. Now, have your partner attack you with a circular punch. As soon as you see him move, lunge forward and extend both arms upwards towards his face, hitting with a fist or palm strike. Unless he is extremely fast and you are inordinately slow, you hit him before he hits you. Of course the more alert you are and the more you have practiced, the sooner you are able to see his attack, providing you with more time to respond. Blast forward as soon as you see his shoulder movement, or if he is an amateur, as soon as he pulls his fist way back like John Wayne.

Although you have a decided advantage by starting your blow from centerline, that doesn't mean you can go out for coffee before you respond. Concentrate on exploding forward as soon as you recognize his attack. If it helps, imagine you are a sprinter, running the 100-yard dash. You get ready, set, and then wait for the official to fire the starter pistol. It's the same here (except if you hear a real gunshot, you better run faster than any sprinter). Try to be ready mentally to advance the instant you see the window of opportunity.

Practice 1 or 2 sets of 10 reps on each side.

Next, have him throw a straight punch as you respond with the exact same technique you did against the circular punch. This one is a bit trickier to pull off, but with the right timing, you can divert his attack to either side of your punching arm as you drive forward and land your attack. Try getting a slight upward angle in your arm to help "cut" through his punch.

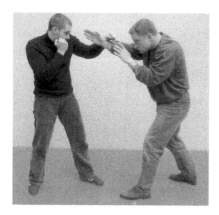

Your opponent attempts to jab, which you deflect from your centerline stance, and then shoot in a palm-heel strike with the same hand.

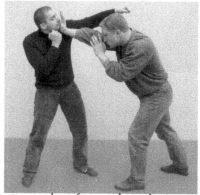

Your timing needs to be precise when moving forward against your opponent's straight-line attack. If you move too soon, it might not work, and should you go too late, you would likely block his fist with your face. Time it perfectly and his attacking arm slides off yours as you slam a powerful blow right into his mug. Many people are afraid that their fist will smash knuckles to knuckles with the attacker's fist. We can't really exclude this possibility but it's unlikely to happen if you time your move right, which is the whole purpose of this drill.

That said, better duck your head a little at first until you get the hang of it.

Practice 1 or 2 sets of 10 reps on each side.

Control his spine

A key element of centerline is that it passes through your spine and, equally important to remember, it passes through your opponent's spine, too. Your objective is not only to control your spine, but his, too, which benefits you in these ways:

- It greatly hinders his ability to attack since he needs to rotate or at least move his spine to deliver techniques.

- It's difficult to impossible for him to use his footwork when he lacks control of his spine.

- You force him to have to deal with your control over him before he can do anything to you.

- Inexperienced fighters won't recognize that you control their spine via the centerline and typically try to keep powering through, though their best efforts fail. This gives you time to counter them and even laugh about it.

- An experienced fighter recognizes the trap and tries to escape, making him too busy to attack you.

- By controlling your opponent's spine, you buy yourself more time to do whatever you have to do to him. With more time available, you don't have to depend on speed or muscle, but rather effective techniques.

Let's look at two examples of controlling your opponent's centerline:

- Just as your opponent begins to attack, lunge forward and execute a hard palm push high on his chest at his centerline. With your body mass behind the push, combined with the momentum of your lunge, his balance is broken and he is momentarily helpless to do anything about it. His priority is to stay upright as he flails his arms. Without retracting your pushing arm, launch a front kick into his groin. *Practice 1 or 2 sets of 10 reps on each side.*

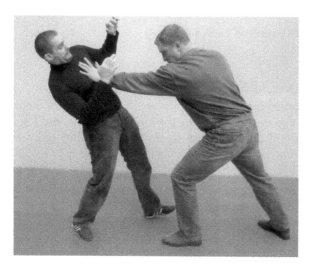

Disrupt your opponent's attack with a push high on his chest at his centerline, and then slap kick his groin.

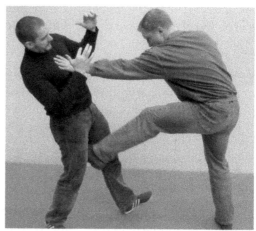

- Duck under the attacker's wild swing and lunge into him, jamming his upper arm against his body. Lean into it to make sure he can't push you backwards. Focus your pushing energy straight into his centerline so he is forced to shift his weight to remain in balance. He has three options: spin, turn or retreat. If he spins around for a spinning elbow or backfist, step a little to the side if needed, and shift your controlling arm to stop him, leaving him vulnerable to your other arm. If he turns and reorients toward you to attack with his free arm, hit him before he brings his other weapon into play, and if he retreats, follow and hit with whatever technique fits the timing moment.

 Whatever he does, your control of centerline gives you a window of opportunity to do whatever it takes to end the fight. Your reaction time is fast, too, because you know that he can move only one of three ways. What if he doesn't take one of the three options and just stands there? Well, think of him as a breathing punching bag and hit him at will before he changes his mind and tries to escape. *Practice 1 or 2 sets of 10 reps on each side.*

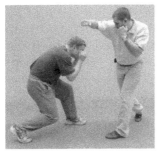 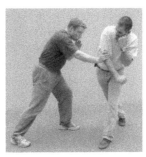

Duck under your opponent's punch and press his arm to jam him.

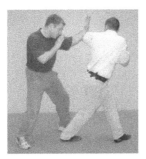

If he spins block it and counter.

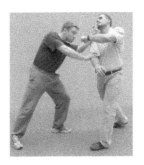 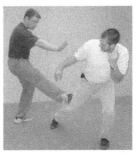

If he tries to hit with his left, keep jamming and counter and then kick his leg as he retreats.

The boxer's stance

Since boxing is primarily a fighting art for sport, most boxers use a classic stance where they position their arms on each side of centerline to protect their heads. This is because they wear 12- or 14-ounce gloves, making it nearly impossible for anyone to jam a fist into that open centerline; the gloves are just too big to pass through. Over the years, consequently, many sport boxers have neglected protecting their centerline (though we are happy to report that this is beginning to change). That wasn't the case in the old days.

Look at pictures of the bare-knuckle boxers of the early 1900s. Their hands are almost always near or on their centerline and, in many instances, their stance and hand position are similar to those found in many Asian martial arts. Also, the way they fought back then was closer to what you see in a street scuffle, as opposed to the way boxers fight in the ring today. The sport of boxing has evolved over the years, but those early champions can still teach us a thing or two. For example their punches were designed so that their bare knuckles held up to all the pounding they did on their opponent's hard skull. They accomplished this by aligning their fists in such a way that the punch would shoot straight and on centerline. This accomplished three things:

- It ensured that their straight punches followed the shortest route from their on-guard position to the target.

- Punches were executed with the fighter's bodyweight behind them, which made it less necessary to rely on raw muscle for power.

- Upon impact, the fist was supported by a good biomechanical structure. It dissipated the force by flowing back into the fighter's fist, wrist and arm, reducing the chance of injury.

Check out these two photos. The one on the left shows a "modern" boxing stance, while the one on the right depicts one that is "old school." Notice the difference in the two pictures as to how the hands are positioned in relation to centerline.

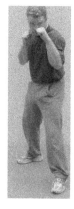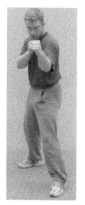

Now look at these pictures. The first one shows a jab executed from a modern boxing stance. This version is most often delivered as a quick, snappy blow meant to sting rather than hurt. Its power is derived from the acceleration of the punching arm, as opposed to one that has the fighter's bodyweight behind it. Fighters who favor the jab tend to use a lot of footwork as they annoy their opponents by zipping in and out of range. Though this can sometimes be a useful technique for self-defense, we feel it is more appropriate in a competitive context.

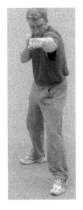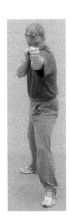

In the photo on the right, the technique looks a little different when the centerline concept is involved. First, the body is twisted completely so that more power is added to the blow than is in the sports-like version. Add footwork to launch you forward and your entire mass is behind the punch. In many ways this version is similar to the basic thrust in the art of fencing. With these additional elements, what was a relatively weak punch now has knockout power.

Practice 1 or 2 sets of 10 reps on each side.

If you have been training in the noble art of boxing for a long time and haven't been using centerline, it will take some tweaking and adapting before you feel comfortable with this modification to your jab. Once you get it, though, you will possess a powerful new street weapon, and jabbing in this fashion in the ring will surprise and hurt your opponent, especially if he doesn't know the old school boxing tricks. Typically, jabs are used to setup other, harder techniques. Consequently, a lot of fighters, even street fighters, shrug off their opponent's jabs as inconsequential; some don't even care if their opponent lands one because they feel they can just absorb it. But a jab fired from the centerline isn't average; it's a face re-arranger. If you are lucky enough to face a guy who disrespects the jab, change his mind with your well-trained centerline blow. After he is dazed and confused, you have ample time to follow up with any other technique of your choice.

Works with other techniques, too We use the jab as an example, but you can apply this centerline alignment for all your straight punches. It works whether you strike high or low, whether you fight with a left or right lead, and whether you attack with the lead or the rear hand. What is important is that you think centerline, and then twist your body and arm so they are completely aligned on it.

Perhaps the most interesting facet of using centerline when punching is that it reduces all excess motion, all telegraphing. This alone affects the timing of your attacks because they instantly become faster with less baggage to drag along. This makes it less likely that your opponent will perceive your attack in time to react.

Demeere once worked out with a classically trained boxer, beginning with a few drills and then hand-pad training. But not until they boxed a few rounds in the ring did Demeere experience the unsettling timing of those centerline punches. His friend just stood in place waiting for Demeere to step into range, and then would hit him in the nose with a jab or cross. The man's fighting stance was twisted in such a way that his fist on his lead arm was completely aligned with his elbow and shoulder, masking when it would strike out. Then it would suddenly snap forward without any preparation at all. It wasn't that the techniques were extraordinarily fast, but that they seemed to come out of nowhere as there was no perceptible preparation in their launch. One moment the boxer was standing still and the next moment Demeere was eating his fist.

Train to make this work for you in your fighting stance and even in your I-don't-want-to-fight stance. Combine it with good footwork and you will surprise even yourself at how much power you have, especially with your jab.

Your fighting posture

There are almost as many fighting stances as there are fighters. We are talking of course about how and where you position your hands, arms and feet as you face a threat in the ring or on the sidewalk. Some stances are practical and some aren't. Actually, "stance" is a bit of a misnomer as the word often conjures a frozen posture, which is never a good idea unless you are the designated school BOB, the assigned punching mannequin for the day. But until a better word comes along, stance will have to do.

There are a few minor differences in the stances and postures used in sport fighting and real fighting.

Differences and similarities

When sparring in class or in competition, you tend to move around sooner than you would in most street confrontations. The referee or teacher says go, and you immediately begin moving about in the usual sparring dance of bobbing, weaving, and moving in and out of range. In the street, however, there is often an exchange of words first, a little cursing, some posturing, toss in a dash of pushing, and then the actual clash. While most real fights end within seconds, some do last longer, and with those it's not uncommon to see the two moving about as fighters do in sparring competition. However, it's important to keep in mind that just as some competitors explode forward the moment the ref gives the command to go, some street encounters go from 0 to 60 in a fraction of a second, too. In both cases, any semblance of a stance is nonexistent. For now, let's assume that you have a second or two to get into a fighting position.

A basic stance

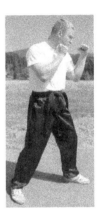

Here are a few thoughts on establishing a basic stance, one that gives you the most for your money timing-wise, and one you can add to or delete from depending on your needs. To begin, think boxing stance: feet a little more than shoulder-width apart, knees slightly bent. Your body leans slightly forward at the waist and your fists are positioned on each side of your face, cheek level. Your chin is pulled in a little with your forehead forward, so that you look out from under the ridge of your eyebrows.

Keep your guard up

When full-contact karate came punching and kicking into our homes via television back in the 1980s, we quickly saw that some of the traditional ways of doing things didn't hold up when the opponent wasn't pulling his blows but was actually trying to send the other guy to Sleepville City. For example, a fighter who fought with his arms hanging down at his sides was quickly dispatched by a spinning heel kick upside his head. When he awoke 15 minutes later, his corner man was usually heard to say, "Uh, maybe next time you better keep your hands up, champ."

More and more fighters are finding that a high guard, similar to a boxer's, works well against most opponents. If you know that your opponent is a kicker, you can drop either hand a little so you can quickly block or check his legs. With your hands up along your cheeks and your forearms in front of your body, you present fewer targets and fewer timing opportunities for your opponent to exploit.

Speed-wise and timing-wise, your high guard allows you to shoot straight punches on a direct line into your opponent's face, punches that are much harder to block than those that come up at an angle from your hip or solar plexus. Should he lower his guard just an inch, shoot a straight-line punch or palm-heel right into his pouty lips. As just discussed in "Centerline," this is superior to your hands held in a low-guard and having to punch at an upward angle.

A high guard also enables you to block a tad faster, especially blows to your waist and higher. From this position, you only have to move your hands a little to swat aside a high punch, or move your forearms in or out to block an attack to your body. The faster you block, the faster you are able to take advantage of the opening, the timing moment, left by your opponent's attack.

Side stance vs. quarter stance

A fighter favoring the side stance quickly discovered in those early full-contact karate fights that his weapon capability was limited. Yes, yes, we know Bill Wallace fought that way, but he and a few others were rare exceptions who got away with it. Those who were more mortal found that to keep from being knocked silly, they needed to use the classic quarter stance with all their weapons upfront and ready to go. In today's competition where so many full-contact tournaments allow hard kicks to the thigh, the side stance would not only be weak defensively, but would position the fighter's legs right there to be abused.

Strong side forward?

Some fighters fight only with their strong side forward, like Wallace and Bruce Lee. While the argument for it makes sense – you place your strongest side closest to the target to ward off incoming blows and counter with fast power – it also makes sense to be versatile, to be able to fight equally, or close to equally, on both sides. If you train only with your right side forward and a street thug whacks your right elbow with a board, or cracks your right kneecap with the point of his boot, you are in trouble. When you practice on both sides, you are more versatile and have a side to use should you get hurt. Timing-wise, you are better able to react to a window of opportunity, no matter what side is forward. Versatility means you never have to let an opportunity pass just because you didn't have your best weapon forward.

Move or pose?

Have you seen any of those old black and white samurai movies from the 1950s and 1960s? Although they are wonderful movies full of noir and incredible sword fighting, they depict the combatants standing motionless before one another, each with his sword in an on-guard position, each waiting for the right moment. Legend is full of tales of samurai standing frozen for two days waiting for a timing opportunity. That was fine back then, but nowadays we lead lives that are far too busy to do that. Who has two days free to stand in a fighting stance? In these modern times, we need to get the battle over quickly.

We're joking, but the point is that you never want to stand motionless.

Muhammad Ali introduced constant movement to the boxing world at a time when many boxers held their ground and only moved their arms a little. Ali danced like a butterfly, stung like a bee and got his opponents to make errors that he happily exploited. This is exactly what you want to do. Now, if you are 25 years old and weigh 165, you can hop all over like a bunny rabbit, but if you are an older fighter and weigh 200 pounds plus, you can only move around so much before you become fatigued. Christensen, who is older than dirt and weighs 200, shuffles his feet about and keeps his upper body, including his arms, in constant motion. Although he isn't hopping up and down like some tournament fighters, this still works to camouflage his attacks and allows him to take advantage of timing opportunities. It really doesn't matter how you move as long as you move, because: *Motion from motion is harder to detect than motion from stillness.* Remember that.

Say you are standing motionless facing your opponent and he accidentally moves his lead leg into range. Think of it as a timing opportunity handed to you on a golden platter. But when you go to kick his errant leg, he scoots back out of range. He wasn't even aware that he had allowed his lead leg to wander into range, but when he saw you move to kick it, he caught on and made his escape. New scenario. This time you are moving your arms around a little and shuffling your feet. Your opponent misjudges the distance and steps into range without following up with an attack. But you do. As a quick as a blink, you pop a hard roundhouse kick into his thigh and follow with head hits. Your opponent didn't perceive your leg kick because its launch came from continuous motion.

Putting it all together, you want a stance that permits you to stay moving, keeps your targets covered, and allows you to fight with equal skill on both sides, all while allowing you to explode on any timing opportunity foolish enough to present itself to you.

Weight, stance and limb positioning

Your personal fighting stance or on-guard position is a matter of preference based on trial and error. Here are a few additional elements to examine how you might apply them to your own needs and capabilities. There are no right or wrong ways to this, only ways that are inappropriate depending on the situation. For example, sometimes you might want to use a deep stance when stability is called for, then a high stance when fast mobility is in order. As we discuss weight, stance and limb placement, we encourage you not to hold on rigidly to what you are used to, but experiment a bit with these ideas to see what works for you and what doesn't. If you like this material, you will have added a new trick to your repertoire. If you don't like it, at least you will have an understanding of it and can recognize it when an opponent uses it against you.

Weight distribution and stances   Human beings are bipeds. They keep their bodies upright and balanced by moving their two legs in coordination with their upper body movements. Some of these movements are overt and others are imperceptible. Anytime you stand in place, your balance is continuously on the job. When standing seemingly immobile, your legs are busy fluctuating the weight distribution from 50/50, 49/51, 48/52 and so on. The precise percentages are determined by a number of factors:

- The width of your stance: A horse stance is wide and stable whereas a cat stance is narrow and requires a tad more balance.

- The position of your upper body: leaning forward puts more weight on your front leg and less on your back one.

If you just had a "Well, duh!" moment, congratulate yourself. While weight distribution is supposedly basic knowledge, even experienced martial artists make mistakes. Unless you train in a variety of different arts, you get used to moving and standing in a specific way while fighting. A karate fighter moves differently than a kung fu practitioner; a capoeria fighter is far more mobile than a muay Thai fighter, and so on. Each martial art has its own way of doing things and this includes weight distribution. There is nothing wrong in general about how these various fighting arts move. Problems arise, however, when it comes to the specific demands of a situation.

Inexperienced fighters, whether sport or street oriented, often fail to use this knowledge. What happens all too often is that a fighter seizes a timing opportunity and lands a successful blow, say a right hook punch, but then continues to hit with it though it's no longer possible to do so effectively. Though he was in good balance the first time, he is now leaning too far forwards or backwards for his second and third hook to be effective. Instead of using another technique to pursue another timing opportunity, he desperately shoots that hook again and again in hopes that it will land.

This is often due to a lack of fighting experience, a problem of not understanding weight distribution and stances. A more experienced fighter would know that instead of using the hook punch again when he is leaning too far forward, it's more effective to fire off a kick from the back leg. He knows this is preferable since his front leg is already supporting most of his weight and he doesn't have to take time to shift his position to prepare for another hook. Timing is knowing what to do and when to do it based on your weight distribution. Knowledge is:

- Understanding weight distribution makes you faster without having to use additional muscle contraction.

- Controlling how and where you place your bodyweight improves your timing as it allows you to use the best technique from wherever and however you find yourself when a timing moment makes itself available.

- Automatically shifting your weight or changing your stance because you know that what you need to do isn't possible from your current position.

Full and empty

In some fighting arts, a person's weight distribution in a given stance is referred to as "full" and "empty." In a forward stance, for example, your lead leg is full, meaning it's supporting more of your weight than is your back leg, which is empty since it's supporting less of your weight. It's the other way around in a cat stance. Whenever a leg is full, it's your main support pillar, the one keeping your body from falling down. As such, it's relatively hard for you to step with it. You can, but it requires muscular effort, and the deeper your stance, the harder it will be. It's much easier to simply move your back, empty leg.

Think of your full leg as your body's stabilizer, a pillar that can absorb energy and keep you in balance, especially when you are pushed, pulled or hit. Think of your empty leg as the mobile one that can move freely and do whatever it wants without taking time to shift your weight from it.

All that is quite simplistic, so let's muddy the waters a little. Rarely is the weight distribution of a stance 100 percent full for one leg and 100 percent empty for the other. Your stances and footwork change continuously as do the percentages of weight distribution on your legs. It's important to think of full and empty as concepts to help you understand what you can do at any given timing moment in a fight, but also remember that the situation changes constantly. The trick is to stay alert to the needs of the moment, ready to change the instant a window of opportunity opens.

Different fighting arts might use the same stance yet distribute the weight differently. As we both reverse punch, Christensen demonstrates a classical karate front stance and Demeere (top) shows a tai chi front stance.

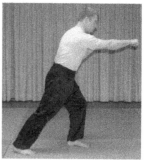

Christensen's stance (which, by the way, he doesn't use but is doing it here for demonstration purposes) is firmly rooted low and wide, back upright, his power coming from a sharp rotation of the hips and a solid base. His upright body makes it easier to add torque to his technique but it also makes the weight distribution fairly even, roughly 60 percent in front and 40 percent in back. The drawback to this is that Christensen needs to push off his back leg if he wants to follow his opponent when the punch knocks him back. This isn't impossible, but he will have to use considerable muscle contraction to do so, which will cause him to be slightly slower than the same action from the tai chi stance.

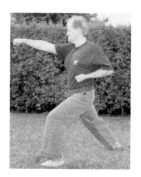

Notice that Demeere's tai chi stance is much higher and that his back leans into the technique to form a straight line with his rear leg, making a weight distribution of roughly 95 percent in front and five percent in back. This helps in generating power for his punch by shifting his weight towards the front leg as he attacks, instead of using hip rotation as the main source of energy, though it's still an option. Since leaning forward places more weight on the lead leg, it's easier to use the back one for a follow up kick or to move in for the kill with a quick step. In either case, Demeere's back leg can move much quicker and with less effort than can the rear leg in the classical karate stance. The main drawback in the tai chi stance is that it lacks the stability of the other.

Know your stances Both are good stances, but the issue is to understand how the differences influence what both fighters can do from each of them and, more importantly, how it influences timing. With this in mind, evaluate your various stances as you train and determine which techniques are the easiest to do from whatever position you find yourself in. Ask yourself which moves are the most logical to execute and what do you need to do to go from an offensive move in one range to a second move in another range. The greater your understanding and the better you are physically at this, the faster you will seem to your opponent, even if you aren't moving all that fast. This is because you spend less time between techniques. As self-defense instructor Marc "Animal" MacYoung says, "I don't spend time *preparing* to attack. Every move I make is an attack." If you can do this, your attacker will think he is fighting a whirlwind as you rain blows on him from all angles. Refer back to the drill "Statue." It's a versatile one that teaches many things, one of them the ability to pick the right technique given the stance you are in at that moment in time.

Limb positioning

Tactical limb positioning is another tool you can use to make your opponent's life miserable. It won't alter your timing as such, but it will change your opponent's perception as to how you are timing your moves. With careful limb placement, there is a difference from how you normally execute your techniques, though it's really more about how you chain them together. This will be clear in a moment.

Shortening the timeline

When most people think of how a punch or kick moves from its beginning to its conclusion, they see it in terms of prepare-punch-retract or prepare-kick-retract. Here is another timeline to help you get a visual of this.

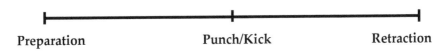

| Preparation | Punch/Kick | Retraction |

Consider a kick. The novice fighter sets up the moment, launches the kick, and returns his leg to his initial fighting position. Then he executes another technique. More or less, that is the standard way of doing things, especially in competitive fighting where judges like to award points for nice, clean movements. The problem is that it takes too much time, relatively speaking, to complete a technique to where he can move on to the next one, a wasted moment in which a savvy opponent can hit him in the nose.

Begin your follow-up sooner One element that makes for an experienced fighter is his ability to combine techniques quickly. Consider boxing's basic jab-cross combination. Where a beginner, or an experienced fighter who has picked up some bad habits, fully retracts the jab before he launches the cross, a better fighter begins retracting his jab at the same time he begins shooting the cross. In the case of the aforementioned kick, the better fighter starts his follow-up backfist *as* his kicking leg returns to the floor, and then hits with it at the same time his foot touches down.

Attack from any position   Say you want to counter with a left hook to your opponent's ribs but your elbow is too high after blocking his high roundhouse kick. To punch, you would first have to bring your elbow down a tad, an action that wastes precious time.

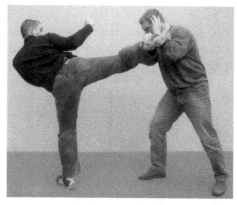

You block his high kick but find your left elbow is too high to counter punch the ribs without first lowering it.

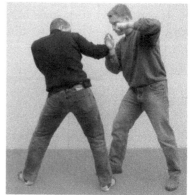

As you found in the Statue drill, it's faster and more efficient to attack from wherever your arms and hands happen to be the instant a timing moment appears. No overt preparation, just an explosive launch from where they are at that moment. It's easy to do, though it does take practice to do it right. Here is an example: Block that same high roundhouse kick by raising your elbow next to your face. Now, don't retract your blocking elbow, but instead straighten your arm and scoop/grab his leg as he begins to retract it. It's as if your block was preparation to grab his leg. By not making that excess movement to cock your fist, you increase your overall counterattack speed and amaze your opponent at what he feels was perfect timing at grabbing his leg. Which it was. From there you can do a variety of throws and takedowns.

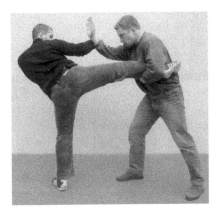

A faster response is to scoop his leg and execute other counters.

Practice 1 or 2 sets of 10 reps on each side.

Expansion and compression Let's take it one more step and look at an interesting fighting concept found in many martial arts systems. Kuntao/Silat expert Bob Orlando calls it "Expand-compress-expand," and in tai chi chuan, it's called "Combining-closing-and-opening movements." By whatever name, it allows you to make the most out of each move you make because no matter where your limbs are when a timing moment appears, you can hit without overt preparation and wasted movement. The objective is to blend each technique into the next one in such a way that the last technique is preparation for the next. This achieves two things: It eliminates excess preparation and eliminates retraction on the timeline. What is left is the attack. Here is how Bob Orlando describes it:

"Before demonstrating this technique, it is helpful for you to recognize and understand another concept that is used here -- the concept of expansion and compression. This is not magic; it's not even uniquely Indonesian, but it is an extremely worthwhile concept to understand. To begin, ask yourself, "What is a punch?" (A rhetorical question, right?) No, seriously, what is a punch--what is it mechanically or kinesthetically? Setting aside the obvious, a punch is at least two things: It is an extended arm and it is simultaneously a chambered elbow. Now, along that line of thought, what is an elbow strike? It is two things: a folded, contracted, collapsed, or compressed arm, and it is also a chambered hand. What this means for the martial artist is that the actual execution of some movements (parts of techniques) simultaneously readies, prepares, or chambers others--like some imaginary double-barreled gun where the act of firing one barrel automatically chambers a round into the other."

Think of this as shortening the timeline into just one element: the attack itself. The other phases have completely blended into the attack, resulting in a much faster execution of your technique. Timing-wise, it's about knowing what technique to use and when to use it.

By striving to shorten your timeline to the absolute minimum, you continuously push your opponent into a new OODA loop. Since each move is an attack, he becomes overwhelmed quickly, increasing the likelihood of your success. Take a look at these examples.

- Take the initiative by shooting a right palm-heel straight into your attacker's face, snapping his head back and forcing his upper body to lean back. Without missing a beat, grab his shirt with the same hand and pull him straight into a knee to the groin. Then as you pull back your knee, execute a right hand push to drive him onto the floor.

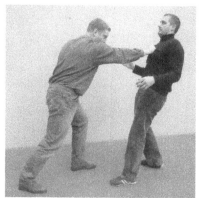
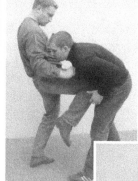

After striking your opponent's face, grab his shirt with the same hand to pull him into a knee strike and push him down.

- (*This is probably too long to be practical, but it's a good one to get a feel for the concept*) Block your opponent's right swing with your left hand as you step into him. Then shoot your right forearm into his neck to force his upper body to lean backwards. Immediately pull back your right arm, clawing the side of his face, and with the same hand punch downward into his stomach, doubling him over. From there, snap your right elbow into his exposed chin and finish him off with a hard, right palm strike to his chest to knock him away from you.

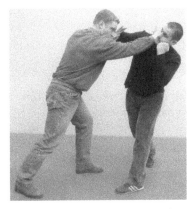

Block your opponent's left punch and shoot out your right forearm to his neck.

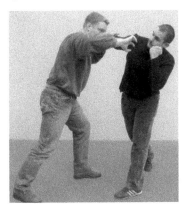

Claw his face on the way to . . .

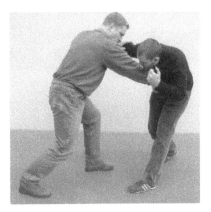

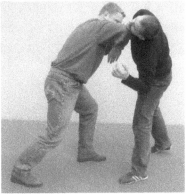

. . . punch his stomach, and then snap your elbow into his jaw. Knock him away from you.

- Step into your attacker's right punch and simultaneously block it with your left as you hit him in the face with your right palm. Without pausing, hit him in the body with a left straight punch while you retract your right hand for cover, should his attacking arm still pose a threat. From there, shoot out that right hand again to punch him in the throat.

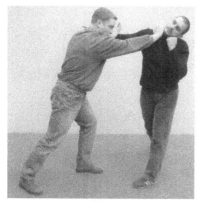

Step in and strike a right palm to your opponent's face.

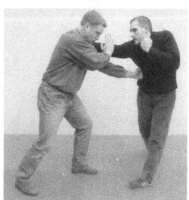

Retract your right hand as you punch his body with your left ...

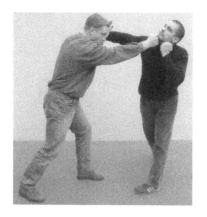

and then check his arm again with your left as you punch his face with your right.

- Your opponent attacks with a straight punch. Sidestep it and knock it downward a little so you can grab his wrist. Use your other arm to soften him with a hard backfist, while pulling his wrist toward you. This breaks his balance and dazes him at the same time, providing you with a window of opportunity to step in and take him down with a hip throw.

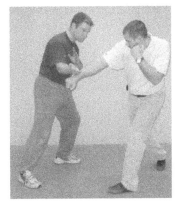

You sidestep your opponent's right punch . . .

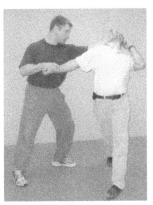

grab his wrist and yank him into your backfist . . .

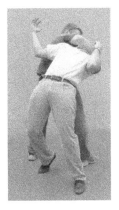

and then step in for the throw.

In each of these examples, you move from wherever your attacking limb happens to be into another attack. Sometimes you follow with another technique using the same limb, while other times, you switch to the other arm. Which one you use depends on the attack and how well you can chain things together. What is important, though, is that you no longer prepare or retract your attacks by accident or habit. Each movement you do is deliberate and because you know what technique follows best from wherever your limb happens to be after the last attack, it appears that you are running on a sort of automatic program, one that is efficient and seemingly fast. A punch becomes preparation for a grab, a grab turns into a push, which positions you to deliver a rib-breaking body blow. Your opponent feels as if it's raining blows and because he is busy in his OODA loop, he doesn't have time to counter. As soon as he feels the pain of one attack, the next one is already landing, and so on until he is lying on the floor whimpering in pain. Because you now chain your techniques with limb placement in mind, he simply doesn't have sufficient time to stop you from beating him.

Slow? Improve your timing

You are standing there, a picture of innocence when a street-creep suddenly begins woofing at you. You try some verbal judo (see Chapter Three), but it fails. You try to get away, but he has blocked your avenue of escape. You have but one option left: go through him. You notice that for the few seconds he has been in your face he has repeatedly opened and closed his right hand. Then he pulls back his right shoulder. You are about to get sucker punched. Without looking at your watch, you know it's time to hit him with a pre-emptive strike. It's all about timing, now. You have been given a perfect moment, one where he is going to react too late to your surprise attack and fall unconscious to the ground.

You launch a perfect palm-heel jab to his chin, but he slips it with ease and counters with a blindingly fast and vicious hook punch to your exposed ribs. Okay, that hurt. And now you are in an all-out brawl with a guy much quicker than you.

Having to fight someone faster than you is the stuff of nightmares. Whether it's in the street, your martial arts school, or the ring, facing a speed demon is never fun. Most fighters train hard to develop their optimum speed to keep pace with these guys. But what about those people who are naturally slow because they have a preponderance of slow-twitch muscle fibers or some other physical malady that limits their speed of movement?

As discussed earlier, fast-twitch muscle fibers are responsible for explosive movement. If you are unfortunate enough to have only a low percentage of them, you will never be "naturally fast," a term used for people who, without any training whatsoever, can be even faster than trained fighters (we hate those guys).

People termed "naturally slow" are the exact opposite. They excel at sports like marathons and triathlons, activities where extreme speed is less important than endurance. It's fairly easy to determine if this is you, though it costs a bit of cash and some pain. It necessitates that a doctor take a small muscle sample from you and analyze it for composition. If you don't want to spend the money or you are as scared of doctors as we are, it's easier to simply go over the following checklist. The more you answer "yes" to these questions, the more likely you have mostly slow-twitch muscles.

- Have you always performed poorly at sprinting, the high and long jump, and weight lifting with heavy weights?

- Can you jog for an hour straight, even if you haven't trained for it?

- Is it hard for you to counter when sparring, though you see the opening and can visualize the right technique?

- Are you always getting hit when sparring?

- Does it seem like you are always slower than your sparring partners?

- Have you tried a variety of speed drills but haven't improved?

If just one or two of these bullets apply to you it doesn't mean you have predominantly slow-twitch muscle fibers. But if three or more apply, it's likely you do. Now, don't despair and put your head in a gas oven, as not all hope is lost for you as a fighter. Even if you aren't as fast as these other guys, you can still beat them. You just have to train more and outsmart them with good timing. Here are a few things you can try.

Feinting

Feinting is a strategy that has endured the test of time for the simple reason that it works. From open battlefields across the centuries to the back alleys of today's metropolitan cities, fighters have used feinting to help them defeat even superior foes. The concept of a feint is to do just enough of a technique - punch, kick, stance change - to deceive your opponent into thinking that you are going to do the complete movement. Then, just as he responds to your partial technique, you initiate another to score.

Far too many fighters throw feints that aren't believable and, therefore, fail to get a reaction from their opponent. To avoid this, your feint must be a real technique, albeit a partial one. Do it convincingly enough, by including body movement and even facial expressions, and your opponent will react, leaving him vulnerable to your second technique, the real attack.

A good feint can even break your opponent's concentration and send him into a new OODA loop when he realizes suddenly that the technique he reacted to is no longer there. Kuntao expert Bob Orlando says, "Feint something that causes him to react, then pounce with something else once he commits to defending the feint. The best fighter I know is not particularly fast. However, he possesses an almost uncanny ability to hit his opponent whenever he wishes, especially when he sets him up with believable feints."

Many people either feint poorly or time their feints improperly. Here are some points that will help your feinting skills be as good as the best fighters.

- **Feint only when you have a follow-up to do.** As ridiculous as it sounds some fighters throw a beautiful feint and then don't do anything else. A feint all by itself is useless and can leave you open and vulnerable. A feint is meant to create a timing moment, a window of opportunity. If you don't act upon it because you aren't sure what to do, it will go away and you just might end up spitting out dirt from your opponent's shoe.

- **Be at the right distance for whatever technique you plan to follow with.** If you are too close or too far from him, whatever opening you create will be long gone before you hit it. If you want to smash him with your roundhouse kick, don't fake with an elbow strike since you will be too close to land a kick. Likewise, don't fake with a partial sidekick when you plan to follow with a headbutt. This should be obvious but we see it happen all the time. Also know that if you feint from too far outside of your effective fighting range, your opponent realizes immediately that you are only feinting and will be alert for more.

- **No two people react the same way to feints.** Some will be as jumpy as an often-kicked dog and others will just look at you like a cow staring at a passing train. A good amount of fighting experience, no fighting experience, fatigue, alcohol, drugs, and even stupidity all affect how people react.

- **It takes experience to know the right amount of motion to elicit a response.** Do too little and your opponent won't notice and won't respond. Do too much and it's as if you executed a real technique that missed. Do it too far away from your opponent and he just laughs at you. Experiment to find what works best in a variety of situations.

- **Don't use too many feints in the street.** Fighters in the ring have several rounds to feel each other out, experiment with feints, and explore offensive and defensive techniques. In the street, however, fights usually last only a few seconds so there isn't always time to dance around and throw fakes. Besides, you don't want to prolong the confrontation any longer than you have to. Most often it's best to feint only once or twice and then end the fight with your follow-up.

Training your feints for the street

Square off with your partner and run trough your entire arsenal of feints using your head, arm, kicks, grabs, footwork, and even shouts. Your partner should give you honest feedback. If he feels your feint isn't convincing enough, he tells you so. Now, don't take it personally and come back at him with, "Yeah, but your mama's a thief." Learn from the critique and strive to correct the problem.

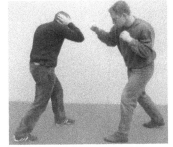

Here are a few tricks for you to try. They are simple because our fighting philosophy is simple. It's already hard enough on the streets without getting complex in your self-defense.

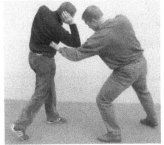

Switch levels of attack   Fake an attack to your opponent's legs and when he moves to block, hit him in the face. The bigger the difference in the levels, the harder it is for him to defend against your follow-up attack. If you can't hit at extreme levels, do less. Fake a head punch, and when he dodges, slam a hard punch into his liver.

Practice 1 or 2 sets of 10 reps of each combination

on both sides.

Switch sides   Feint to one side of his body and when he moves to protect it, hit his other side. For example, throw a left hook at his face and when he lifts his guard to block it, fire off a hard right palm strike to the other side of his face. Feint a punch to his right side and then land a kick on his left side.

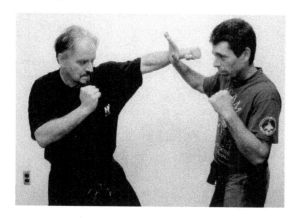

Launch a hook punch at one side of his face and he just might drop his guard so you can whip in a powerful slap.

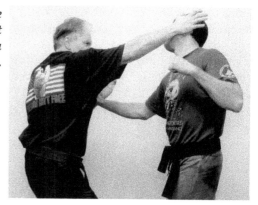

Baiting

Your opponent has plenty of time and opportunity to counter when your punch or kick is slow to get to its target. Obviously, this isn't good for you, but it's something you can turn to your advantage. It's not easy, as it requires a good sense of timing and a strategy based on baiting your opponent to force him into a certain reaction, one you are ready to act upon. Once he commits to his reaction, he can't react as quickly to your new attack, though your basic speed is slower than his.

Say you notice that your fast opponent always drops both hands to block one of your kicks. Good. Next time throw a kick you can do with little or no leaning. Just as he drops his fast hands to block or smother your kick, hit him in the ear with a backfist. Though he possesses great speed, it's nearly impossible for him to change gears and successfully block your high blow.

You can use virtually any reaction you can coax from him to land a solid hit that leaves him gasping for air. Your imagination and technical skills are the only limitations here, so feel free to experiment.

- Bait him with a punch and when he reacts, kick him.

- Bait him with a kick and when he reacts, punch him.

- Shoot in for a takedown to force him to lower his guard and block you, and then hit him in the face with a palm-heel strike.

- Step on his foot so he either leans back to retract it, or he ducks in pain, and then backfist his nose.

Do 1 or 2 sets of 10 reps on each side.

As you and your training partner experiment try to keep it simple. Though complexity might work in a tournament setting where you are fighting against another trained martial artist, in the streets, where your opponent has probably never seen your fancy karate set-up, he just might force you to eat a garbage can lid. Keep it simple in the asphalt jungle. That said, if you have been working on a couple of basic baiting techniques that you can perform well under a variety of circumstances (keyword: variety), and you have tested them under pressure in training, then they just might be street applicable.

Lead him into a trap   Sometimes even a good feint isn't going to help you against that super-quick fighter. If you fear this is the case, consider setting a trap for him by taking the idea of baiting one step further. Instead of creating an opening by attacking him, give him an opening that is too good for him to refuse. Let's say you expose your face to him. When he goes for it, you have a nasty surprise waiting for him, one that will be hard for him to block since you put him abruptly into a reactionary mode, back in a new OODA loop. Even if he is much faster than you, the action/reaction principle is at play here, meaning he has to mentally and physically stop to react to your new attack. That gives you time.

Limit his attacks Earlier we discussed various factors that affect reaction time. In short, the higher the number of attacks your opponent has for a given situation, the longer it takes you to pick the best response. If in addition he is faster than you, well, it was nice knowing you. Just kidding. Here is a way to use that against him.

By baiting your enemy into attacking a specific opening that you deliberately gave him, you reduce the number of attacks he can use to just one or two that are applicable to the location of the target. For you, defending against one or two possibilities is much better than trying to defend against six. Fewer choices for you increase the speed of your reaction time, enabling you to overcome your speed disadvantage. Here is an example.

Say you know from your opponent's previous matches that he is quite skilled with a large arsenal of hand attacks. So as the two of you dance about, you drop your right, rear hand, which opens a path to your right ear. As long as you face him straight on, you reduce his response choices to a circular attack: a left hook punch, a right backfist, a circular kick. By reducing how he can attack, you also reduce your blocking choices to one that simply protects the right side of your head. Fewer choices for you mean a greater response time. You simply lift your right arm and easily block his circular attack. Since your opponent probably didn't have time to figure out the cleverness of your strategy, of your mental game, he is left thinking that you suddenly became alarmingly fast.

Though there is no absolute guarantee the attacker will fall for the trap, or use the specific technique you want him to, it's our experience that more often than not, he does. Under the stress of a real fight, people tend to keep things simple: They see an opportunity and they go for it. This means that when you are in that back alley and present the attacker with a nice clear opening, chances are good that he will take it. However, if you overact or in some other way get sloppy with your baiting, he might see the trap and use it against you. This is the inherent risk of this strategy (and the inherent risk of hanging out in alleys). If your opponent doesn't fall for it, he just might set you up for a fall. Here are some additional points to consider.

- It takes confidence and a calm mind to pull off a good trap. If you are fearful and tense, it will be hard to respond to the attack you lead him to.

- Leading is often used by older, more experienced fighters who rely on their fighting experience and good timing, rather than sheer muscle-power.

- Trapping works for young or novice fighters, too, as long as they train hard on it and keep it simple with punches and kicks they are comfortable with. For the street, they should leave their fancy, jump spinning kicks in the trunk of their car.

Grab your partner and experiment with a few ideas to incorporate leading. Many fighters find that this works well in combination with the scenario training discussed elsewhere. Once you have a feel for leading your training partner into a trap, try working it into stress-inducing scenarios. If you can implement an effective trap under stress that approaches what you might encounter on the street, you are on the right path.

Here are a few trapping ideas for you to try, especially in stress-induced scenario training:

- Drop both of your hands to make an obvious opening to your face.

- Raise your guard more than normal to expose your midsection.

- Drop or raise just one hand to reveal an opening on one side of your face.

- Allow your lead leg to stretch out as a ruse for him to kick or stomp it.

- Lean slightly forward or backwards, as if a bit off balance, especially against a known grappler who will try to push or pull you further in the off-balanced direction. (Tip: When he pulls you, move into him quicker than he expects and mow him over with your counter.)

- Stick your chin out a little. Don't be blatant about it, as an experienced fighter won't be fooled. It's best to combine the action with some verbal taunting, which works to enrage the inexperienced fighter and bait him into taking a swing. There is some risk here for you in that you might get so caught up in your verbalization that you fail to duck or slip his punch. This is why it's good to practice trapping with stress-inducing scenario training.

- Assume an I-don't-want-to-fight stance and tell him that you don't want to fight. When all indications from him are that a fight is imminent, turn your palms up and move your arms away from each other to give him a clear path to your centerline. Most fighters will use a straight-line attack right at your midsection. (Tip: Step to the side as you parry his attack and counter with a roundhouse kick to his stomach.)

Practice 1 or 2 sets of 10 reps on each side of all the above listed techniques.

It takes time and effort to know how much (actually, how little) opening to give your partner. Too much and he gets suspicious and might not go for it. Too little, and he might not notice. Ask your training partner to give you feedback as to how you are doing. Practice before a mirror, or in front of a video camera. The more feedback you get, in whatever form, the better you are going to be at trapping.

In all of these traps, and any that you devise, it's critical that you counter at the earliest possible moment: As soon as he steps into range to react to your trap, or as soon as he shifts his weight in whatever direction to deliver his response, that is the instant you hit him. Remember, you are trapping him because he is faster than you, so you want to hit him at the earliest opportunity.

Timing when you are already fast

"I feel the need...the need for speed," Tom Cruise in *Top Gun*.

Okay, so you skipped all the earlier pages about how to apply timing when you are slow because you aren't slow. (Actually, you should read them anyway because the tips there will make you even faster.) You rarely have problems landing blows, you block like greased lightning, and you launch attacks with blistering speed, all without even trying. Perhaps you are naturally quick and have always excelled at sprinting, jumping and all physical activities requiring explosive speed. Your moves are quick as a wink from the first time you learn something, and your classmates have to work twice as hard to be only half as fast as you. You are one of those predominately fast-twitch muscle fiber types (who we would hate if you hadn't been so nice and bought this book). As such, you have an enormous advantage in martial arts training, competition and self-defense situations.

Don't be like Mohammed Ali

First, thank your parents for the blessing of speed, but keep your ego in check because you aren't unbeatable just yet. Look at the man considered by many as "The Greatest," Mohammed Ali. He was a gifted and unconventional boxer with incredible hand speed, great reflexes and nimble footwork, all of which gave him the ability to dodge punches, while moving away from his opponent and countering simultaneously with a flurry of jabs, crosses and hooks. Though there is more to his success than just that, his awesome speed was an underlying factor in his fighting strategy. As Ali got older, however, his speed started to desert him (combined with other problems), and his fight game began to suffer. Since his speed had been a cornerstone of his fighting style, once it diminished, his overall performance decreased and he began getting injured.

Can there be a downside to speed?

Just because you have awesome natural speed doesn't mean you get to win every match or real fight. If it can backfire on The Greatest, it can happen to you. In fact, your speed might be the biggest reason you lose. Here's why:

Problems in the ring   It's common to see young athletes with perfect genetic makeup rise to the top of their sport at an early age. They beat nearly all their adversaries with little or no effort. They have natural talent, natural speed and seem to be born to play that specific sport without a lot of hard training. It's a sunny day for them, but it's about to rain on their parade or, more specifically, it's about to rain when they hit the big leagues. At that level, fighters have a similar physical make-up, combined with skill developed from hours of training. At the highest level, it's that one, hard-training fighter wanting it the most who goes home with the gold. Those young, talented fighters who didn't train hard because they took their genetic potential for granted, and who didn't understand that they have to increase their training 10-fold to face equally gifted, but better-trained fighters, will have to deal with the agony of defeat. For them, their natural speed has hindered their technical, tactical and psychological evolution.

Problems in the street   Though this problem is apparent in the sport side of martial arts, it's no less of an issue in self-defense. Should you rely too much on speed to beat your attacker, you risk failure somewhere along the line. One day, you face an opponent who has a solution to your lightning strikes. If it's a good day, you only get the stuffing beaten out of you, but if it's a bad day, you get worse. It doesn't even have to be that much of a fighter to do it, since you do most of the work against yourself for him. Instructor Frank Garza says this:

"If you rely only on speed, then you can't take advantage of the openings that happen after a well-placed hit, because if you're in a hurry, you hit targets that aren't always open, which exposes you to getting countered. On top of this, very few people can hit hard and hit fast. I think timing is more important than speed. I know my hands are pretty fast, but what makes me even more effective is that I have the patience to wait for the openings."

If you have great speed, it's tempting to just launch a salvo of attacks and wait for your opponent to drop. Sometimes this works, but sometimes it doesn't. Don't become so dependent on your speed that you neglect to time your techniques to fit neatly into your opponent's openings. A wiser course of action is to use your speed to strike vulnerable parts when they are exposed, instead of banging on a closed guard or using risky techniques you can do because of your speed.

Kickboxing great Bill "Superfoot" Wallace had kicks clocked at over 60mph, an incredible speed that many opponents felt most painfully. Wallace has said that he liked to kick people in the face from close range, a distance where a punch would be quicker and easier, just to embarrass them and drain their morale. This works in the ring, as it certainly did for Wallace, but out in the streets, it's a risky way to defend yourself. Picking a more difficult technique when an easier alternative is present is not good tactically, and it's potentially disastrous timing-wise. Instead, it's better to concentrate on taking advantage of mistakes your opponent makes, as well as using one or all of the ideas in the list below.

No matter how fast you are, it's always risky to put all your eggs in one basket, even if your speed is a huge ostrich egg. Relying on one factor, as superior as it might be, won't solve every problem you encounter. You are better off developing additional skills. Instructor Garza gave us a great example of a student of his:

"I had a student named Roger who was very fast with his hands and feet, and frustrated many people. Since he didn't have power to go with the speed, his kicks and punches didn't hurt me, but they were annoying. I figured out how he telegraphed his punches and kicks and at what range he liked to throw them. With my timing, I was able to use his speed against him, as I knew what he was going to throw and how he was going to throw it. When he did, I had a kick/punch waiting for him.

"One of my other students, also a grappler, was getting frustrated fighting Roger. So I told him to just go in and pick him up and slam him to the mat. He did, then Roger didn't want to play with him anymore. Now, Roger was a great student, but because he only had speed, he couldn't hurt too many people, just make them mad enough to where they wanted to go inside and hurt him."

Now that you are thinking about not relying solely on your speed, here are a few ways to improve your fighting skills, particularly your timing, using your great speed as a foundation. Think of you speed this way: It isn't your entire chain, but it is an important link.

- **Perfect your technique** As just discussed, many naturally fast fighters tend to compensate for their lack of technical expertise by relying on sheer speed. In doing so, they ingrain improperly executed but fast techniques into their bodies. Then when their speed diminishes with age, they are left with bad techniques that can be nearly impossible to correct since they have been doing them wrong for decades. Don't let this happen to you. Train hard to have good techniques now so that not only are you a better fighter today, but you will still be a good fighter when you get older. Know that you can't go wrong by always working on your basics – reverse punch, jab, backfist, and the four basic kicks, front, round, back and side. Strive for mastery of form, speed and power.

- **Set up your power shots** A good, fast lead-hand jab is like a lightning strike, whereas the reverse punch, the cross, is considerably slower. This is because the jab is close to the target and involves minor body movement, compared to the reverse punch that comes from the more remote rear hand and requires a complex coordination of stepping, twisting of your hips and upper body, and traveling a greater distance. The biggest difference lies in the power potential of the two. The jab is mostly a set-up or distraction for a follow-up technique, while the cross is a heavy hitter that packs lots more punch.

It's just possible that with your natural speed that you can get away with launching a powerful cross with less preparation than slower fighters or, if timed right, without any preparation at all. As a result, your speed enables you to land hard, fight-ending punches without having to first set them up with a jab or backfist. How do you know if you have the speed to do this? Practice. Experiment. Especially against fast opponents. Know your capabilities and you are half way to victory.

- **"Double tap"** This is a firearms concept where you fire two quick rounds into the same target to inflict more damage than a single shot. The same concept can be used in your empty hand training. When you spot an opening and the timing is right, ram not just one fast attack into the "hole," but two fast blows. You have the speed for it, you have the opening and the perfect timing moment, so enjoy yourself and thump him twice. For example, duck a circular punch to your face and shoot a fast left-right punch combination into your attacker's gut, instead of just the left or just the right. Or, after you duck, use your left forearm to drive your opponent into a wall as you double punch his solar plexus with your right fist.

- **Combinations** For our purposes here, let's call a combination a sequence of more than two blows, more than the double tap just discussed. When slower fighters try to hit three or four rapid blows, their opponents can often counter them halfway through the combination. But with your natural speed, you are well into your third or fourth attack before your opponent has the time to react. In a full-contact match or a street confrontation, your well-placed powerful blows are likely to overwhelm your opponent before he can even muster a counter-offensive. This is the whole purpose of using longer combinations: to force your attacker back into the OODA loop, thus reducing his time to recover or adapt to the ever-changing angles of attack.

Attacking in combinations isn't the same as doing a wild flurry of uncontrolled punches and kicks. Throwing good combinations is like playing pool, where one shot sets up another, though in this case, one hit sets up a timing moment for another. To do this, you must construct your combinations strategically and experiment in training to find the ones that suit you and yield the best results. Here are three:

1. Change your levels of attack by going high, low, and then high again.

2. Attack one side of your opponent's body to create an opening on the other side.

3. Hit his body in such a way that his body moves right into your next blow.

Practice 1 or 2 sets of 10 reps on both sides of all three combinations.

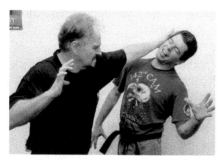 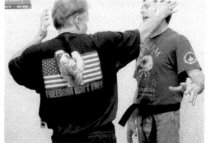

*A hard slap on one ear knocks his head into your next
circular attack on his other.*

With each of these, and any others you devise, you must be cognizant of all available openings, all windows of opportunity created by your blows. For example, say the street thug suddenly leaves his head and groin open. *Bam, bam,* you hit both as quick as a wink, forcing him to twist hard to the side, exposing the side of his closest knee and a vulnerable ear. *Bam, bam,* you hit those a half beat instant after the first two hits.

- **Beat him to the punch**   Your super speed makes you an ideal candidate for using pre-emptive attacks, a combination of good timing, deceptiveness and speed. (Be sure you are justified legally to hit first or you are going to be lying on a steel bunk staring at a small window high on your cell wall.)

  A thug makes it clear that he is about to hit you. Lean back with your hands up in your I-don't-want-to-fight stance, your lead leg extended slightly toward his groin. With your upper body leaning away, you look farther away than you really are. When the bozo looks over to one of his pals to see if he is getting a laugh, you seize the moment to pop your size 10 shoe into his groin. *Practice 1 or 2 sets of 10 reps on both sides.*

- **Outguess him**   This tactic is ideal for a naturally fast fighter, though it still requires keen timing and experience at recognizing specific attacks. Whenever your opponent throws a punch, one that you perceive an inch or two into its launch (this is where keen timing, a sharp eye and experience come in), attack him immediately in the opening his technique creates. For example, the instant he launches a right reverse punch, his right flank is open, which you strike happily with a counter as you block. If he uses a left roundhouse kick, sweep his defenseless right support leg. *Practice 1 or 2 sets of 10 reps on both side.*

Know that every attack has a weakness, one you can use against your aggressor as a result of your awareness and speed. While many fighters can see the opening, they aren't fast enough to attack it. Spend time learning the weaknesses of the most common attacks, learn to recognize the early stages of them and then have fun blasting your attacker in the resultant weak spots.

Don't rely only on your speed

Just as you would never depend on one technique to save the day in every situation, it's critical that you don't rely solely on your great speed to defeat every opponent. Speed is wonderful and it's fun to be fast and it's fun to watch a really fast fighter. But it can also be your downfall, especially when dealing with an experienced technical fighter. It's important that as a student of the martial arts and self-defense that you strive to maximize your chances of success by employing every possible factor. Be grateful for your speed but train hard to use it to its fullest by developing all your other skills and assets to serve you well right now, and in your later years when your speed begins to slow.

Age, injuries and speed

The years teach much which the days never knew.
~ Ralph Waldo Emerson

The good news and bad news about age and injuries

• The bad news is that, yes, you lose some speed as you age, but the good news is that with continuous training you won't lose that much and you will slow the ticking clock.

• The bad news is that Father Time has a way of reminding you of your foolishness as a young person by haunting you with old injuries that can inhibit fast movement. The good news is that if you are careful and cognizant of your training, nutrition and rest needs when you are in your teens, 20s, 30s and 40s, you will limit the number of injuries that add drag to your movements in your later years.

• The bad news is that if you are now a teenager or in your 20s, and you are hard on your body and live only for now, you are in for a rude awakening when you turn 40 or 50. If you are particularly hard on yourself, you might even get shaken awake at 30.

Co-author Christensen began training in karate in 1965. As a 19-year-old, he had no concept that he would still be training today at 58 years of age. Though he was quite abusive to his body in those early years, there are only two or three injuries that still affect how he moves now. He feels fortunate that his 30-year-old broken kneecap and his 13-year-old injured forearm tendons are the only major injuries that affect his speed today. All things considered, it could be a lot worse.

If you are 18 years old, it might be hard to think about doing things now to prevent problems 30 years into the future. But you must. Unless you get run over by a careening gasoline truck, you are going to be around 30, even 40 years from now. Keep that in the back of your mind when you awkwardly push up those extra-heavy weights, and keep that in mind when you decide an aerial somersault would be a nice touch in your kata. Not only can injuries sustained from poor training and extreme training come back to affect your martial arts in years to come, they can also affect your training right now. Bottom line: Train smart and you will train long and healthily.

About the passing of time

As athletes, we tend to deny that the passing years will affect us, but our denial doesn't change the fact that we *will* change. There will be a degree of decline in physical capacity, but happily it can be slowed. As just discussed, the first step is to prevent debilitating injuries. The second step is to keep training. All of us lose around one percent of our physical capacity each year after age 35, mostly in the area of cardiovascular (aerobic capacity), musculoskeletal (muscle and bone mass), and metabolic function (assimilation and elimination). It happens to elite martial artists who train everyday, to people who train only once or twice a week, and it definitely happens to people who don't train at all. But, continual training, maintaining a good fitness level, and eating a healthy diet can all help to minimize the loss.

Another difference between men and women

Males peak in strength and speed between 20 and 25 years of age, and females peak around 18 -- unless both sexes participate in a long-term training program. By including weight training, aerobic exercise and martial arts training, you can keep improving until your mid 30s. From 35 on your strength declines slightly, then remains at the same level for 20 years or more – but only if you train. It's all about continuous training.

There are exceptions to these numbers and you can do much to slow the process with proper training and good diet. It's not uncommon for hard-training martial artists in their early 40s to be told by their doctors that they have the physique and internal system of a person many years younger.

Many trainers say that you will never again be as fast as you are in your 30s since speed tends to decline steadily from there. Co-author Christensen says that this common belief isn't what he has found. He was in his late 40s when he wrote *Speed Training: How to Develop Your Maximum Speed for Martial Arts*. For the eight months it took to write the book, he drilled continuously on the many exercises and training concepts discussed in the book. He didn't work on them with the expectation of getting faster, because at that time he held the belief that it wasn't possible at his age. Instead, he worked on them so he could better describe them in detail. To his happy surprise, however, he discovered his speed improving; with some moves, his speed increased many times over. Now, would he have developed greater speed if he was 30 years old when writing the book and doing the exercises? Of course. But his improvement at 48 was pretty darn good, too. And he never complained.

At the age of 57, Christensen made a training video titled *Speed Training: Secrets of Developing, Increasing, and Exaggerating Your Fighting Speed*. Even at this age, he discovered his speed improving as he practiced those last few months prior to the shoot. He plans to do a project on speed when he is in his 60s to see if improvement is possible even at that age.

Since speed deterioration is primarily caused by a loss of that one percent lean muscle mass per year after 35, the more muscle mass you have when the decline begins, the slower you lose it. Don't misread that into thinking you have to be a competitive bodybuilder, because too much mass inhibits and slows movement. You just need well-developed muscles that are applicable to the martial arts.

Use your muscles or lose them. Weight training is your friend. Dynamic tension training, where you pit one muscle against another, and free-hand exercises - push-ups, weightless squats and so on - are also your friends. It's all about training consistently and progressively to stimulate your fast-twitch muscle fibers.

Continual training as the years pass will buy you additional time. Since the human body is complex and so many variables can affect your life (such as that aforementioned careening gas truck), it's impossible to say how much time you can buy. We do know that it's quite common for a consistent athlete to maintain the strength that he possessed in his 30s well into his 50s and even 60s.

Think fast

Many top martial artists agree that an important part of the effort in training for speed, some believe a large part, is to *think* you are fast. Yes, think it. Christensen concurs. He says that as he worked on *Speed Training* he found that a good percentage of his increases came as a result of thinking so much about speed during the writing project. As he physically worked on the drills and speed concepts, his mind was continuously thinking: *I'm getting faster. My hands are quick. My kicks are lightening fast. I'm moving ever faster and faster. This exercise is making me faster.* There is definite power in continuous positive thinking.

There are limitations to this. If you are homelier than a mud fence, well, all the positive thinking in the world isn't going to change that.

About timing skill

When asked if older martial artists can possess good timing, knife-fighting expert Michael Janich said, "I sincerely believe that older martial artists naturally compensate for their diminished strength and speed by developing higher levels of timing. Morehei Uyeshiba's extraordinary skill during his later years was, in my opinion, largely due to his keen sense of timing."

Aikido instructor Larry Kwolek also referenced the aikido founder. "If you look at the videos of O'Sensei Morihei Uyeshiba or any of the older senior teachers now, they don't move so very fast, but their timing is exquisite. My teacher in Japan, Shoji Nishio Sensei, is 74 this year and still practicing after over 50 years of judo, kendo, iaido and, of course, aikido; his timing is amazing. So I think if you have been training for a while your training will increase to the point of where you are still able to anticipate the attacker despite your age.

Veteran karate champion Dan Anderson agrees that older martial artists can have good timing: "Absolutely. In fact, as your physical skills deteriorate with the aging of the body, your timing does not have to. Timing is a decision of *when* coupled with the ability to *recognize*."

Christensen used to have a student who was the same age as he. The man always waved off Christensen's encouragement to work extra on his speed, aerobic capacity and flexibility, saying, "You have all those attributes because you have been working on them for many years." The man missed the fact that there was another student in the class, a man who had been training for only two years and was happily making progress in his speed and power, a man 62 years old, six years older than the student who wouldn't listen.

Actually, the man did have a point in that there was no way he could catch up to his teacher's experience, but then that isn't why he should have been training anyway. Trying to be better than someone else is never a healthy goal. His goal should have been to compete against himself, to train to be the best he could be. If he had opened his mind to this objective, he would have improved beyond what he could have ever imagined. Consider these thoughts about age and timing.

- There is no way the new older student can kick as high and as fast as that annoying 20-year-old black belt. But with practice the older fighter can time his slower low kicks to slam into the kid's groin with great prejudice.

- There is no way the older fighter can match the younger one's quick backfist, but by keeping a tight defensive posture, the older fighter can block the fast strike and time his counter to land as the backfist is retracted.

- Where the younger fighter can just go hit, hit, hit all day, the older person has to think, think, think.

The older person does much of this already in other phases of his life, from his business dealings to how to best clean the garage without blowing out his back. The martial arts is just one more endeavor where wise thinking, combined with patience and conservative moves wins the day. Watch an old dog and a puppy. The puppy bounces all around the veteran dog, nipping at his legs, zipping in and zipping out, all while yapping and leaping about in a complex, erratic tornado of puppy energy. Then -- *ku-whack!* -- the old timer swats the puppy with a simple paw-heel strike that sends the young one loppy-ears-over-tail across the floor. Some puppies charge back, though others choose to run off and play with a stick. Those who do come back, show more respect.

An older student new to the martial arts should:

- Pay attention to basics: jabs, reverse punch (cross), backfist, hammer strikes, and chops. Stress the basic kicks: front, round, side, non-turning back kick.

- Don't waste your time on non-fighting techniques like cartwheels, tornado kicks, flippy-dippy kicks that have little impact, charging suicide punches, and so on. Keep it simple and keep it real.

- Develop a sound defense. Master blocks and covering.

- Learn to read telegraphing: shoulder movement, twitching hands, twisting foot, facial expressions, tugging at the pants, a chambering fist and others.

- Learn to react to your opponent's momentary distraction. Hit when he looks away, when he changes his stance within range, lifts his leg for no reason, or overreacts to your fake.

- Learn to fake without over committing your weapons. Use hip fakes, facial expressions, shoulder twitching, and short hand fakes of only two or three inches.

- Develop the ability to evade and hit as your opponent executes an attack.

- Develop the ability to follow and hit as he retracts his blocked attack.

- Study how other fighters stalk their opponents, set up attacks, leave themselves open, move within their stances, and any other aspects of fighting that you can exploit. While all fighters have their idiosyncrasies, all have much in common, too. The more you know how fighters fight, the more knowledge and experience you bring to a confrontation, whether in class or in the street.

Master Sang H. Kim in his wonderful book *Martial Arts After 40* answers the question, *"Aren't you getting too old for martial arts?"*

Kim said: "No. Martial arts can be practiced as long as, if not longer, than just about any other physical pursuit. In fact, martial artists often get better, not worse, with age. Perhaps you are not as fast or flexible as the younger students in class. Perhaps you don't recover as quickly from your workouts or you are bothered by new aches and pains that you easily shook off when you were younger. These are minor obstacles when you consider the benefits that come with age. The wisdom to slow down, to see the lessons in every class, to mentor younger students, to laugh at the macho posturing and go your own way, to discover yourself from the inside out. That is what martial arts after 40 is about; a journey of self, a discovery of the boundlessness of your mind and body, working as one, expressing your inner joy and wisdom."

So there it is. Don't fret because you can't kick head high or punch as fast as that kid over there. Instead, concentrate on what you *can* do and how to make it even better.

Know yourself

So it is said that if you know others and know yourself, you will not be imperiled in a hundred battles; if you do not know others but know yourself, you win one and lose one; if you do not know others and you do not know yourself, you will be imperiled in every single battle.

~ Sun Tzu, *The Art of War*

A man and a woman are sparring in class, and the man notices that she continuously drops her lead hand. "Yes!" he says to himself, "Next time that happens, she's going to taste a little of my glove." Thirty seconds later she drops her lead, giving him a nice opening. He fires off his relatively slow backfist, which she blocks easily and counters with a taste of *her* glove.

In this case, the male fighter knew he had a slow backfist, a problem he had been working to improve for several months. It was getting quicker, but obviously not quick enough. After sparring for five minutes, he detected that his opponent systematically lowered her lead hand, exposing a path to her head, but he didn't factor into his intelligence gathering that she lowered her lead for only a fraction of a second, not long enough for him to score with his sluggish, though improved, backfist. Bottom line: He failed to know his opponent and himself, which caused him to miss-time his technique and lose the moment.

Do you know yourself? Do you know which of your techniques are slow, which are mediocre and which ones are quick as a blink? If you don't know, why don't you? Hey, it's your job to know. It's good information to have when sparring in class, when competing in a tournament, and when fighting in the dark, dank streets. Self-knowledge is critical when you want to take advantage of a window of opportunity.

Co-author Christensen had a minor bout of polio when he was a child, which affected one leg. While there are kicks he can do fine with it, there are others that he doesn't do as well. He knows this about his leg, so when an opening presents itself, almost begging to be kicked with the leg in question, Christensen either hits the opening with another personal weapon or simply allows the opportunity to pass. He knows it's better to let the moment go than to try to score with a weak technique that might get blocked and countered.

Christensen also suffers from a tendon injury in his right forearm. Twenty years ago, he used to offer a dues-free month to any student who could block his super-fast, right backfist -- and he never had to pay. Today, he would never make such an offer because that tendon has slowed his backfist and, on some especially painful days, prevents him from throwing it at all. Since he understands this, he doesn't use it when an opening appears unless the student is a slow underbelt or a black belt having a poor day. There are plenty of other techniques he can use instead or he simply lets the opportunity pass. Since he knows this about his right backfist, he doesn't make himself vulnerable by throwing a slow one.

Training log

In our book *The Fighter's Body: An Owner's Manual*, we harp endlessly on the importance of maintaining a training log. Besides noting data on your diet, sleep, martial arts training, and weight workouts, you should also note information about particular techniques. Write down those that are especially fast, those that need concentrated work or, if it's a physical problem, those that will never be top notch.

Those you deem fast, drill on them in a variety of timing situations to develop confidence and an understanding of their utility. Those you have noted as needing work, devise a training regimen to bring them up to par. Those that are relatively poor because of a physical limitation, think about how you can camouflage that reality and be stronger in some other way. Bill "Superfoot" Wallace has a poor right leg, the result of an old injury. But for years he brought home the gold in competition by kicking solely with his left, albeit a mighty fast left.

Now, there is no room in the martial arts for negativity. Yes, you have determined that your, say, right sidekick needs work, or that your bad right hip will always limit your right-legged kicks, but you must not think of this as a weakness. If your kick just needs work, think of it as a training goal. If there is a physical problem, think of it as something you need to work around, just as you do when sparring a long-legged opponent or a particularly crafty one. Don't go, "Oh poor me," but go, "I'll be strong and fast in spite of my hip."

Gear the fight toward your fast techniques

If your lead-leg roundhouse is so fast it's invisible to the naked eye (yeah, you wish), consider setting up timing moments where you can use your speed. If you know your opponent drops his lead hand for a fraction of a second, be ready with that awesomely fast backfist of yours. Consider faking with your bad right hip to get your opponent to drop his guard, and then hit his opening with a fast left kick.

It's all about self-knowledge: taking advantage of your fast techniques, understanding your slower ones, and always thinking positively. It's self-knowledge gained from training with partners, doing lots of solo training sessions, self-analysis, and making notes in your training log.

How to use timing to increase your power

Hit him as he moves forward

Now, don't skip your weight training workouts just because we show you how to immediately increase your power. Keep pumping the iron. It's been our experience training thousands of students over the years that those who train with weights are miles ahead of those who don't. They have better control of their bodies, their coordination is often better, they are able to put more weight behind their blows, and once they learn to stop flexing and apply their power strategically, they are capable of delivering incredible impact.

Whether you lift weights or not (please do), here is a little timing trick that instantly adds power to your punch or kick. There is nothing complicated here, as you simply use your opponent's forward momentum to meet your technique head on. Consider this analogy. You are driving along in your fine-ride at 60mph. When you go to take a sip of your soda, you inadvertently turn the steering wheel to your right and ram smack into a parked car. Okay, that hurt and you are going to have a scar, but there is a bright side. The car you hit could have been coming at you at 60 mph, too. That car's 60 mph meeting your car's 60 mph head-on would really hurt and scar you because the head-on meeting of the combined speeds increases the impact at least two-fold.

Here is how you can do a controlled head-on with a partner. Your objective is to meet his forward advance with your forward advance plus your technique. This can be applied in several scenarios.

- **He moves in at irregular intervals**   There is no planning here; you happen to be moving forward as he is moving forward. However, if you have practiced for such an occasion, you have an excellent chance of beating him to the punch. Tell your partner to lunge in at irregular intervals as you spar. Your response is to explode forward with the quickest technique in your arsenal, usually something with your lead-hand or lead-foot. With regular practice, you can make your response a reflex, an explosive one that beats your opponent to the punch and surprises the heck out of him. *Practice 1 or 2 sets of 10 reps on both sides.*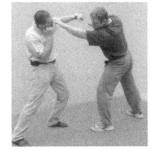

- **He moves in regularly** This is nearly the same as the last bullet except his advance is a bigger part of his fighting style and, most importantly, you know it. Since you have trained in the drill just mentioned, you are ready when he steps into range.

- **Draw him forward and hit him** In this situation, you make a conscious effort to sucker your opponent into moving into your blow. If you know he is a follower, deliberately step back so that he follows, then lunge into him with a punch or kick. Try the broken rhythm concept: Step back, and when he follows don't hit him. Step back again, and when he follows don't hit. Step back a third time, and when he follows with some degree of comfort that you aren't going to hit him -- hit him. *Practice 1 or 2 sets of 10 reps on both sides.*

You and your opponent move in at the same time, but you are first with a quick backfist.

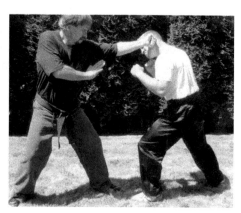

- **Hit a supported target** This concept is strictly for self-defense and it's important that you keep in mind that the potential for serious injury is quite high. The idea is to strike a target when it's positioned against a wall or the floor. For example, when the back of your opponent's head is braced against a wall – he tripped and fell into it or you pushed him there – a blow to his head is going to be absorbed completely. Since there is no place for the energy to go, meaning there is no give, all the power from your palm strike or kick goes right into his skull, with a potential of serious injury. However, when he is away from the wall and his head is not supported, the force of the blow isn't entirely absorbed. This is because the head moves away from the impact, which allows for "energy bleed," meaning, the movement of his head dissipates a portion of your blow's power.

This also applies when it's the floor supporting a target. Say you have knocked your assailant down so that he is, at least briefly, stretched out. To prevent him from getting up, deliver a pile-driving stomp onto his thigh. Since there is no give to the floor and his leg can't move, his thigh absorbs all the energy from the stomp. There is no energy bleed, but there is a lot of terrible, debilitating pain. And limping.

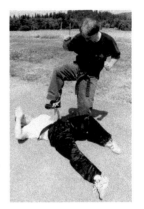

When the attacker's body is supported by the floor, all of the impact goes into the target.

It's not easy to set up a timing moment to hit your opponent's supported limb. It's more likely that the moment will just happen in the course of a fight. That works just fine as long as you recognize it and seize the opportunity to strike. Here are a couple of ways to practice the opportunities just described:

o As you spar, you notice your opponent move just inches away from a wall. When the moment is right, use your forearm to slam him into it, and then use your other arm to launch a powerful reverse punch at his chest, a punch that, if landing for real, would be even more powerful and painful because of the supported target. *Practice 1 or 2 sets of 10 reps on both sides.*

o Execute a slick foot sweep so that your opponent lands on his back. Before he can react with a counter from the ground or attempt to get up, simulate a stomp to his belly, a kick that if not controlled, would feel excruciatingly powerful and painful because there is no give to the target. *Practice 1 or 2 sets of 10 reps on both sides.*

Although not impossible to set up, hitting a supported target is more likely to happen in the course of the fight. When it does, your training enables you to see the opportunity and act on it. And your assailant will think that Hercules thumped him.

Know the power of your weapons

Self-knowledge, that is, knowledge of your strong points, is important when you want to set-up an opponent for a timing moment. Let's say you have an especially powerful right-hand slap. You have trained hard on the bag and have improved both hands, though you are especially fast and strong with your right. Don't try to figure it out; that is just the way your body works.

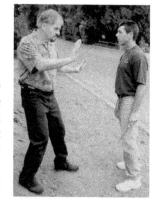

Use your power move

You have been having a bad day and to add to it, you are now facing a man having a road rage fit over some perceived wrong you did when you pulled into the parking lot. He is about four feet away getting worked into a tizzie as he threatens to turn you into corn chowder. During the course of your effort to calm him with verbal judo and deescalation moves - none of which have worked - you notice that he tends to circle to his left, your right. A screwdriver materializes in his hand from somewhere, and he holds it along side his leg. Your hands are up at shoulder height, palms toward him. He has given you no choice but to fight. Just as he takes another little step to his left, your right, you step to your left with your left foot, leaving your right hand right where it was, an action that extends your arm. His step has placed him unwittingly right into the firing range of that nasty slap of yours. Your right arm whips like the lash of a dragon's tail, and your palm makes a loud *splat!* as it flattens and distorts the thug's face.

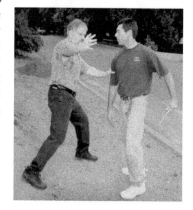

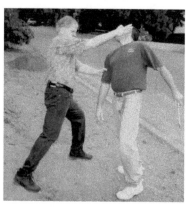

You are trying to calm an irate man when you see a screwdriver in his hand. Quickly step away from the weapon, leaving your open hand where it was as a distraction, then whip it forcefully into the side of his face. At this point you would either control the weapon arm or run.

This worked for you because your instinct told you that bobbing and weaving with a guy armed with a screwdriver was not a good thing, but that ending the confrontation quickly was. Since your careful analysis of your training, both in class and in your solo practice, has shown that you have a man-stopping right-hand slap, and you saw a weakness in your adversary's fighting style, you set up a moment of opportunity for yourself. Life is good.

Here is a technique that doesn't have the same impact power as a slap, punch or kick, but it will have a powerful effect on the attacker. We're talking about the eye poke.

Say your aggressor pushes you backwards with his right arm. Immediately grab his wrist with your left hand and simultaneously whip the fingers of your right hand across his eyes. Now that he is distracted and in considerable agony, move your right hand to help your left establish firm control over his wrist, and step out and pivot your hips to twist his arm. Trap his arm in your armpit and apply pressure at his elbow joint.

Practice 1 or 2 sets of 10 reps on both sides.

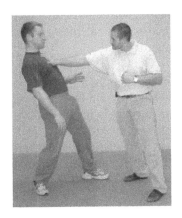
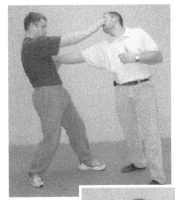

When your opponent pushes, grab his wrist and simultaneously rake across his eyes, then flow into a joint lock.

Use your speed

Say you have a lightening-quick combination, a low sidekick to the knee and forearm ram to the throat. It's one you can do smoothly and with lots of power. Think in terms of setting up the opportunity. Maybe you notice that he steps into your kicking range without doing anything. Set up a timing moment by stepping or leaning back a little so that he follows. As soon as his leg is in range, drive a smashing sidekick into his knee and slam your forearm against his Adam's apple. Then scramble away.

Practice 1 or 2 sets of 10 reps on both sides.

Use your weak techniques

Say your left jab isn't progressing at the same rate as your other techniques. Does that mean you should never use it? Not necessarily. If you have a powerful reverse punch, look at using your jab to force your opponent's hands up and then drive in your power blow. This is a bread-and-butter combination for many fighters, but what is different here is your thought process. You know your jab would be like hitting him with a marshmallow, but right now you don't care. You use it only to set up your man so you can knock him down with a mighty blow from your right.

Maybe you sprained your left wrist in a clash or the street thug cut it with a swipe of his knife, and now it's useless. No problem because you can still use it to set up your power blow. You can fake with it or use it to flip blood from the cut into your adversary's eyes. In this day with all the blood borne diseases out there, people are easily made excitable when blood is tossed into their face, not to mention that it really stings. Take advantage of his panic and pain, and slam your power blow into him.

Practice 1 or 2 sets of 10 reps on both sides pretending to have a cut or sprained wrist.

Caution: Be careful that you don't think so hard about setting up a timing moment for your power techniques that you fail to see other opportunities, or even fail to see that he is setting you up, too. Stay open to every possibility, offensively and defensively as you sucker the guy into your power technique. Remember the concept of an open mind, Mushin, discussed earlier.

Eliminate excess movements

Excess movement is like jogging with a backpack filled with 50 pounds of barbell plates on your back. Excess, by its definition, means more than you need. In fighting, whether play or real, excess movement slows you, tires you and almost always leads to failure. Get rid of it now, every last bit of it. Here are a few ways to do that.

Train before a mirror

There is good and bad about a mirror. If you are so homely you have to sneak up on a glass of water to get a sip, a mirror is a constant reminder of that reality. But if you want to work to get rid of technique-slowing, excess movement, a mirror is a good thing. Recognizing that you are doing big or even little things that encumber your ability to act on a timing moment is a step toward eliminating them. Working before a mirror provides you with constant feedback, more than a teacher who patrols the class and stops for a moment to correct your error and then moves on to the next student, leaving you to slip right back into making that same error again. The mirror provides you with data as long as you stand in its reflection and as long as you know what to look for.

Let's say you have a killer technique but you haven't been able to score with it in class or competition. Say it's your backfist. You can hit the bag so hard that the stuffing *poofs* out of the seams, and your friends tell you that it's as fast as a cat's strike. So why does everyone block it? Could it be that you are announcing its arrival? You might not be verbalizing its arrival – "Ooookay, heeeeere iiiit coooomes!" – but you might as well be because you jiggle your fist, take a deep breath, shuffle your feet and flare your eyes. Your opponent sees all this and moves away, readies his guard, or just simply blocks your attack. It's not that the element of surprise was taken away, it's that it was never there in the first place because you were giving away your intention.

This is definitely a problem, but happily it's not a big one to fix. Stand before a mirror and pop out a few backfists. Ah ha! You notice that you are drawing back your hand and turning your body a little before you launch it. That can be fixed easily by repping out a few dozen non-telegraphing backfists with both hands. Done. Problem's gone.

Right. You wish it were that easy.

Most likely it's still there and most likely there were other problems, too. A mirror is a great teacher, but it's not an absolute. It's quite possible that some if not all of your excess movement is done under the stress of sparring. Even if you think you are a cool cucumber, there is still a degree of stress even when sparring with your old workout pal of many years, especially when it gets competitive. When your stress goes up, your adrenaline heats and your heart rate increases, all of which can make you add extras to your technique that aren't revealed in front of a mirror when you are cool and calm. So while you can easily trim the extras from your moves when there is no stress present, know that they might return in a quick hurry and even bring one or two more with them when you add another human to the scenario, your training partner.

Ask your partner to help

Here is a good solution that works for most fighters. Work your problem technique in front of the mirror, ensuring that you understand exactly what is going on and what you need to do to fix it. Once you have corrected the problem, at least in the mirror, ask your teacher or a training partner to watch you spar to see if it comes back. If they say it did, try to determine in what circumstances it appears and then work to eliminate it. They might also tell you that they noticed you are doing some other things besides what you asked them to look for. Great. Make note of their observations and work to eliminate them as you spar and do reps before the mirror. If you discover that telegraphing shows up only under stress, again ask your partner to tell you when it happens so that you are aware of it and you can make a conscious effort to make it go away.

Here are a few typical excess movements that generally appear prior to attacking, and can be eliminated with feedback from a full-length mirror and a helpful partner:

- Tugging at your pant leg

- Twitching your hand

- Drawing in a sharp breath

- Making some kind of facial expression or movement with your head

- Moving all about and then stopping suddenly

- Shifting your weight off your kicking leg

- Chambering your technique more than necessary

- Looking at the intended target

Once you eliminate these unnecessary movements and have worked to make your attack come seemingly out of nowhere, you will explode like a rocket when a timing moment happens.

The value of experience and how to get it

Understanding improves timing

Even if your body contains mostly slow-twitch muscle fibers, you can still possess good timing if you have more experience and skill than your faster attacker. For example, if you have a pragmatic understanding of distancing, you can beat a faster, stronger opponent, and even do so easily. You know that when he is outside of range he can't use a close-range technique without first closing the distance. While this sounds logical and not particularly brilliant, there are always fighters who try. By understanding this simple distancing concept, your safety zone enables you to apply a well-timed attack should your opponent err. Your experience also reveals itself during those times when your opponent has only a couple of options available to him. Say you force him into a corner so all he can do is strike at you with an elbow or knee. Knowing that those are his only options (knowledge gained from experience), your reaction time and counters will be faster.

Reading about these two concepts or any others is a start, but it doesn't mean you can apply them tomorrow in the heat of battle. You need to work on them repetitively, think about them, apply them against opponents who at first let you succeed, and then progressively put on the heat to make the moment more and more difficult for you. Yes, it can be tedious to practice repetitiously, but the upside is that the more you do it, the more experience you chalk up, the less you need to depend on physical strength and speed to accomplish your objective.

The old adage "Youth and strength will always be overcome by old age and treachery" is true. Many men and women working as police officers, soldiers, bouncers, and even criminals and bullies, have experience earned from violent situations, everything from minor tussles to lethal encounters. Those who have thought about their past encounters, analyzed all aspects of them and *learned* from them, will have gained physical and intellectual experience that gives them a greater understanding of how to apply good timing. At the end of their careers, they retire (criminals and bullies are incarcerated) with a greater understanding of the nature of violence than people who live more peaceful lives. When confronted with it they certainly don't dance around and try to score points, but they do what is necessary to end the situation quickly, knowing first hand just how dangerous any encounter can be. This is easily noticed in smart, older ring fighters. They might not have the speed and explosiveness of their earlier years, but they make up for it with skill and precise timing that has been forged through years of training and experience.

If you are young and full of energy, enjoy it and take advantage of it because it isn't going to last forever. Just be sure to develop precise timing, as it will serve you now when you are fast and strong and it will serve you in the years to come when Father Time starts taking its toll on you.

Street experience improves timing

Research suggests that the action you take in the presence of a real threat - gun, knife, a massive outlaw biker with muscles and skull tattoos - when you have an accelerated heart rate and a massive surge of adrenaline and fear, will stay with you much longer than those techniques you repeat in a less threatening environment, such as when you hit the heavy bag in your garage. The brain remembers what you did in those stressful circumstances and, when those actions help you survive, it holds them hard-wired into your memory.

The more actual experience you have, the more likely it is you will do well next time. But, and this is another big but, there are no guarantees here. Anyone can be taken out by a sucker punch or a sudden attack from the shadows. And there is always the chance that you could be confronted by one of those anomalies who has never been in a fight in his life, but given the right circumstances, can be virtually impossible to defeat no matter what your experience. Look at how fierce a petite, seeming nonviolent mother gets when her child is endangered. She will fight to the death to keep her baby from being harmed.

In co-author Christensen's book *Warriors: On Living with Courage, Discipline and Honor* writer Jerry VanCook tells of a stereotypical bookkeeper-type who had never been in a fight or lifted anything heavier than a chess piece. But upon finding out that his wife was having an affair with a big, burly, martial arts-trained police officer, the bookkeeper beat the officer so severely the man had to be hospitalized.

Critique yourself

Understand that experience has value only if you learn something from it. Analyze what happened - what went well, what went poorly - and use your training to correct the errors and reinforce your good actions. Even those things that you did well should be analyzed to see if there might be an even better response. Sometimes a win is just a fluke (this occurs in martial arts tournaments all the time). Could you have dodged that sucker punch? Would a kick have been better than that punch? If so, which kick? If not, why? That you survived in one piece means you did something right. But it's still important to take that experience and see if you might have done something even more right.

Positive experience gives you an edge by making it psychologically easier to do what needs to be done to win next time. If you performed a specific technique, say a palm-heel to the face, numerous times in real self-defense situations, you know what it feels like to do it under stress. That gives you confidence with it and enhances your skill, at least a little.

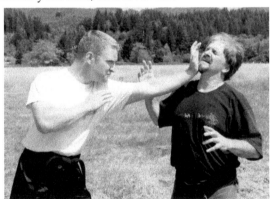

A palm-heel strike is a powerful technique and relatively safe to use against the opponent's boney skull.

To state the obvious, training is only a simulation of a fight. Doing palm-heel strikes in the air repetitiously teaches you the basics of the move, and doing them against a focus mitt or the heavy bag gives you a feel for how the impact is distributed on your hand, wrist and shoulder. Doing them against an attacking training partner gives you the feel of applying them dynamically with a live person. Each phase is important and has value. Still, it might not feel the same the first time you do the palm-heel in the street against a mugger. But you will gain from that experience. Should you have to use it for a real a couple more times, your confidence will increase even more. With training and real experience under your belt, you are more likely to continue to use your palm-heel strike in both, and less likely to miss timing moments with it.

More on training experience

Let's look closer at training as a way to get experience, and continue to use the palm-heel strike as your weapon of choice. Typically, a student stands face-to-face with his training partner and works the strike offensively and defensively. This is fine, but it's not the only way to train the strike. Here are a half dozen more ways for you to respond with a palm-heel:

- Your opponent swings at you as you sit in a chair

- You are on your knees trying to get up and your opponent kicks at your head

- You are on your back as your opponent straddles you and punches at your face

- Your opponent grabs your shoulders from behind, spins you around and launches a surprise attack

- You are in a clinch and before you apply a grappling technique, you have to first find an opening to "soften" him with a palm-heel strike

Practice 1 to 2 sets of 10 reps on each side of all the above.

Play with these ideas for a while and you will quickly discover a host of other situations in which you can apply the strike. A fun way to get creative is to have each student think of a scenario/exercise in which the class can practice the strike: 1 set of 15 reps with each arm, each partner. If your class has 20 students, that makes for 20 scenarios. Rotate training partners each time so that you can work with different body builds and skill levels. At the end of the session, you have a good working knowledge of the palm-heel strike in a variety of scenarios. This all counts as experience because each scenario requires a slightly different way of timing and delivery, adding to the database of information on this technique.

Musing about real experience and training experience

Unless it is your job as a law enforcement officer, soldier or bouncer to confront violence, it isn't smart to go looking for trouble on your own. In fact, it's illegal. You will indeed get timing experience by fighting in bars but it's quite possible to bite off more than you can chew (or the other guy might bite off something of yours). If you win, you could be looking at arrest and/or a lawsuit, and if you lose, well, that can really hurt. There might not be anyone to save you once you discover the nerd you challenged is in fact a seasoned brawler, or he has six other nerdy friends ready to tap dance on your prone body. Violence isn't as glamorous as portrayed on the silver screen. It's frightening to discover that what you thought was going to be a minor scuffle has turned into mortal combat, and that what you do in the next fraction of a second just might determine whether you live or die.

We strongly advise against going to this extreme. It smarter and better to train consistently, realistically, to include drills with stress factors, and to strive to be committed to keep learning and innovating. There are many ideas and training concepts in this book that provide you with experience in general and timing in particular. Combine this information with what you learn from your instructor, what you learn when training alone (Christensen offers a shameless plug here for *Solo Training*), and what you learn with training buddies, and you will acquire a vast amount of experience. Try, analyze, critique, and evaluate. Put some techniques in your "save" pile and toss others in the "trash bin" when you are absolutely convinced they aren't for you.

Modify your training by progressively increasing your speed, power and mental intent to fit the skill and experience you develop. But keep in mind that no matter how good you get, training needs to be kept close to reality. Forget trying to look like Jean-Claude Van Damme and forget running on the sides of walls like Jet Li. Read books, view training videos, learn how different instructors do things, and talk with experienced fighters. Learn from those who have trained hard and have used their learning in the street. From all this, incorporate what works best for you.

Some people say it takes 20 or 30 years of training to become a master in a martial arts style. We believe that it can take more time than that or less than that, as time alone isn't the determining factor. It's about how you train and the depth of your experience and understanding, especially your understanding of the chaotic and unpredictable nature of fighting. Combine these with time to "season" it all, and you have true expertise.

When co-author Christensen went to Vietnam as a military policeman, he had a few years of martial arts training under his belt, but he was still ill prepared for what he was to face. Once there, he was exposed to fights, brawls and riotous conditions on almost a daily basis. His techniques, though powerful and fast, didn't always land as he was used to in his dojo back home. He quickly adapted his training to the reality he was facing and used his growing fighting experience to become more effective. As a result of the high volume and variety of situations he was placed in during his 12-month duty, he got more experience than most people get in an entire lifetime.

Some people with 20 years of training are still mediocre fighters, with little or no concept of good timing, because they lack natural talent, quality experience, or they use training methods that are inadequate or outdated. Possibly all four reasons. Others, who have been training hard and diligently for, say five years, are far superior because they have natural talent, have gotten good experience, and have used superior training methods. While it all depends on a host of factors, one thing is for sure: You can't go wrong when you train hard, think things trough, and keep on learning.

What to do when you can't use footwork

In boxing circles it's often said that a static fighter will never be champion, and there is some truth to this, truth that also applies to winning a street fight. Standing motionless as that doped-up, outlaw biker launches his giant fist at your face isn't conducive to having the same number of teeth to brush tonight as you had this morning. Getting out of the way by bobbing, ducking, weaving and stepping in any variety of directions is almost always preferable to standing in place.

It's one thing seeing a lightweight fighter scoot about the ring like a crazed flea, but it's quite another to see a heavyweight fighter move fast. Christensen says that legendary Joe Lewis, who fought at a bodyweight of around 200 pounds, possessed extraordinary footwork. Watching him move was like watching an image in old flickering movie film. First Lewis was here, then in the blink of an eye he was over there, and then in another blink he was back here. Trying to hit him was like trying to punch a leaf in a windstorm.

Good footwork is imperative for a fighter wanting to take advantage of a timing moment or wanting to create one. While it's more fun to practice tornado kicks and flying scissor takedowns, it's critical that you spend training time and effort polishing your footwork so you can deliver your well-trained punches and kicks, while avoiding your opponent's.

But what if you can't move? What if for some reason, you can't step as freely as you would normally? You might be on a slippery floor. Or your attacker just landed a debilitating kick to your knee, making it excruciating to step. Perhaps you are in a cramped area when the fight starts, such as between two cars or in a narrow hallway. As a cop, Christensen once fought a guy armed with a gun in a phone booth, and he was in several scuffles with resisting suspects in bathroom stalls. Not a lot of room to dance and shuffle in those places. For any number of reasons and situations, you can find yourself in a place where the simple act of stepping is no longer an option. Here are a few things you can try.

Attack first

Say you just left class and you have to walk across a parking lot to get to your car or bus stop. Just as you step between two rows of cars, a street punk appears from seemingly nowhere, cursing and baiting you to get into a fight. He isn't falling for your verbal judo tricks. He is threatening, twitchy and looks to be on the edge of exploding on you. It's clear that you are going to have to fight this bozo. But it's not going to be a walk in the park because the narrow space between the rows of cars limits your ability to step or move about. So hit him first.

As soon as you are certain he is going to attack (his verbal aggression peaks; he clenches his fist; he shifts his weight) you launch a pre-emptive strike. Don't hesitate, don't telegraph and definitely don't threaten him first. Just do it. Hit him when:

- He looks off to the side

- He is in the middle of a verbal threat

- He reaches for something in his pocket

- He changes stance

- He is listening to you tell him how you don't want to fight.

The cramped space isn't desirable for either one of you, but it's worse for the person who is suddenly and abruptly attacked. Therefore, make him that person. Make his life miserable by forcing him on the defensive and moving out of the way of your attack, or at least trying to, without bumping into fenders or tripping over bumpers. He chose the specific location to make it harder for you to defend yourself, but you turned the tables on him by not allowing him the opportunity to exploit the environment against you. Hit him first with speed to take advantage of the moment and then follow with however many blows you need to get away.

Say you land a palm-heel strike into his face just as he is beginning to chamber his punch. It's likely he will stumble back at least one step or even sprawl against the side of one of the vehicles. If he only loses his balance, hit again or shove him to send him to the ground, perhaps banging his head on a fender in route. Getting back up will be hard for him because of the cramped conditions, which gives you plenty of time to run away or land a few solid kicks should he go for a weapon.

Timing that first palm-heel strike correctly is crucial as it just might determine the rest of the encounter. Instead of the thug hitting you, knocking you back, and forcing you to ward off his additional blows in that small space, you took charge of the fight. Because you timed it well, that palm strike provides you with many other timing moments, thus helping you to remain in control of the situation.

The environmental scenario

The best way to train for an attack such as one between cars is to recreate it as realistically as possible. A good place to start is on the mat in your school where you feel more comfortable exploring various fighting techniques and concepts, a place where you can increase the difficulty as your level of comfort with the material grows.

Cardboard boxes   Bring in a few big cardboard boxes and lay them out so they form a narrow corridor as wide as you would find between rows of cars in a parking lot, or in a tight hallway. After you and your training partner position yourselves between the boxes, your task is to determine how you can slam him into them, while not getting tossed through them yourself.

Training in a confined space is somewhat similar to being in a boxing ring for the first time: You feel cramped. This is good because that is what this exercise is for. In fact, don't think of them as boxes but rather seven-foot-high solid walls that you must use against your opponent. By practicing a number of scenarios, you learn quickly what you can and can't do timing-wise when movement is limited. In the end, you will no longer be intimidated by this kind of environment, but rather look at it as just another place.

A narrow hallway   Once you feel comfortable working with the cardboard boxes, try your techniques in a real hallway. Go slowly at first to avoid injuries and don't pick up the pace until you are ready. Too often, students are anxious to try their material at top speed. What is the point if your techniques are sloppy? Take your time to learn and then gradually increase the speed.

- What kind of kicks can you do?

  - Are straight kicks your only option since there isn't enough room for circular ones?

- If your back is pressed against a wall, what kind of punches can you do?

  - The wall prevents you from drawing your arm back.

  - Are circular and downward blows your only option?

  - Will your backfist work?

On steps   Now move to a set of stairs and see how that environment changes things. Footwork is certainly limited, and standing higher or lower on the staircase than your attacker makes a big difference in what you can and cannot do. For example:

- He is two steps below you and his head is suddenly open.

  - Are you within punching range?

  - Are you stable enough to kick?

  - Can you support yourself against the railing and attack?

- He is two steps above you and his groin is open.

  - How can you punch it without losing your balance?

  - Is kicking out of the question?

  - Can you punch his leg first and then follow to the groin with another hit?

- You are grappling on the same step.

  - Can you force an opening to hit without losing your balance?

  - Can you push him against the wall to create stability that works for you?

  - Can you brace your back against the wall or railing?

  - What can you do to send him toppling down the steps without losing your balance?

Slippery surface   First, surprise your teacher with your innovativeness by pouring 20 gallons of grease all around the school floor. We're kidding. We're kidding! Instead, look for a slick linoleum floor and practice in your socks. Think of the surface as wet grass, a mud puddle, snow, or ice as you examine what you can and can't do.

- What can you do to stabilize yourself so you can attack a window of opportunity?

  - Do you really want to try a high kick as you slip and slide around on the linoleum?

  - Do smaller steps keep you more stable than larger steps?

  - Can you support yourself against the wall?

  - Is grappling on the ground an option?

  - How about eye flicks or throat punches, techniques that don't require much in the way of body mechanics?

Try a variety of footware   Running shoes have different characteristics than dress shoes. Experiment to see how your stability and footwork are influenced by the different shoes you wear on different kinds of surfaces. For example, see if boots provide you with a better grip on snowy ground than do running shoes. You probably have a sense of this already, but doing it for real and feeling what it's really like can be an eye-opening experience.

Your training partner should make it realistic

To get the most out of these scenarios, your training partner must be convincing in his portrayal of a bad guy. He should vary his verbal assault so that sometimes he is aggressive from the beginning of the scenario, while other times he slowly escalates as it plays out. This makes it more of a challenge for you to find the perfect moment for a pre-emptive strike, since that moment rarely occurs at the same time twice.

Timing a pre-emptive strike   Begin by facing your training partner between those cardboard boxes as he woofs you and your mother's reputation. This time, look for the perfect opportunity for a pre-emptive strike but only if his words and actions justify it. Just as he moves within your reach, fire off a hard push to break his balance. It doesn't matter what you push – his arms, face, chest – as long as it knocks him back. Lunge forward, spin him around and propel him through the boxes. Since he is off-balance, it will be hard for him to resist.

If you had been standing in a cramped hallway, that same move would have made him suck wall, if you will, and it just might have cleared an avenue of escape for you. Strike him from behind if you want to buy a few extra seconds, and then run for the exit. Remember, the cramped environment limits your footwork, reducing your time to get away. Don't pause to admire your work, because your assailant just might get back up, madder than he was before. Getting away is always a good idea (and looks good in court, too, as opposed to staying there and beating him into the floor) and it's especially a good thing when your environment makes the situation even more difficult. Focus on getting to safety in all these scenarios.

Next, try the same scenario outside on wet grass. With your footing and your training partner's footing precarious on the slippery grass, your push will send him flying, or you will fall down trying, or you both will crash to the soggy ground. Work on that shove to find the right angle and the right amount of energy that maximizes it but doesn't disrupt your stability. Expect it to be especially difficult to seize a timing moment when exploding forward, as the more abrupt your movement the greater the risk to your stability. Try smaller steps and keep your upper body upright, as opposed to leaning over to push or strike him. Are kicks a possibility? Probably not, but experiment to know for sure. Escape as soon as you can but be careful not to fall in your haste.

Let's look at what you can do when the attacker strikes at you first.

Evade the attack

Evading the attack or simply moving it off course is often the best strategy when footwork isn't an option, especially when you are standing on a slippery surface. Though blocking is a good defensive tactic, it requires a stable base to absorb the in-coming energy that slams into your arms. But stability is the one thing you don't have when sliding on ice or slipping in mud, and a simple block is likely to send you sprawling. Instead, it's best to make your opponent miss in hopes that he will lose his balance as his kick or punch fans the air.

Upper body evasion is the fine art of dodging a blow by moving the target out of the path of the kick or punch. To do this well, you need a keen sense of balance and timing, and the muscles of your waist, hips and upper body need to be flexible. Since your stability is poor, jerking your torso about in an untrained manner is just as likely to make you fall over as is blocking your attacker's incoming punch. With practice, however, this can become a trained, instinctual response that allows you to move with a finesse that not only controls your stability, but also provides you an opportunity to counter attack.

Evasion drill Face your partner in a fighting stance and let him attack you, slowly at first but faster and faster as you progress. He uses pushes and hand strikes, since these are the most stable to do under slippery surface conditions. (Few people are stupid enough to attempt a high roundhouse kick when standing on ice. If you are lucky enough to get such an attacker, move out of the way slightly, and watch his head bounce). Whatever he throws at you, your goal is to move out of the way and do so without moving your feet. Bend your knees to lower your center of gravity and shift your weight as you duck to the side, lean away, lean back or twist your upper body. Then counter the instant his blow misses from whatever position you are in. With luck on your side, his missed attack will cause him to lose some degree of balance, making him vulnerable to your nasty counter. Even if his missed attack doesn't throw him off balance, your avoidance of his blow should put you in position to counter. Aim for his eyes, ears, nose and throat, targets that are highly vulnerable when struck and don't require tremendous power and commitment from you.

Practice 1 to 2 sets of 10 reps on both sides.

Deflecting the attack

Say you are in a narrow hallway or a phone booth, and you can't move your body or head to avoid a punch or push. You must deflect the attack. To be clear on our terminology, blocking means you stop the attack, while deflecting means you change the direction it's heading by slapping or parrying, preferably away from you.

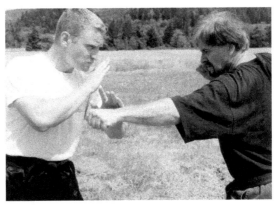

A parry changes the direction of an attack.

The advantage, as it relates to stability, is that you don't have to use footwork, or at least you don't have to use it much. Often, the attacker is surprised by this sudden turn of events and thrown slightly off balance. This is good, but you still need to take advantage of the window of opportunity created by your parry.

Parrying drill   Again your task is to not get hit by your training partner, but this time you deflect his punches and shoves with your hands and arms. Leave your ego at the door and don't rush this phase. Your partner should attack slowly at first and increase his speed only when your skill improves. First practice at slow to medium speed to ingrain the technique as it relates to the timing moment. Only when you are convinced you are ready for faster reps should you kick it up a notch.

The final stage is to counter right after deflecting your opponent's attack. Don't waste time loading up a power blow. Parry his attack and immediately fire a shot, using whichever hand is most applicable, into whatever target he has exposed by virtue of having attacked you. "Open the door" with a quick counter and then follow with additional blows.

Practice 1 to 2 sets of 10 reps on both sides parrying only (If you are new to parrying)

Practice 1 to 2 sets of 10 reps on both sides parrying and countering (If you are familiar with parrying or have practiced the first phase and feel you are ready for this one)

Evading and deflecting

Now let's combine both drills so that you dodge a blow and parry it at the same time. In the first two concepts, the environment dictated which method you use, but in this situation, you can do either. So do both to double your chances of not getting hit. When your opponent punches at your face, move your head to your left just enough to avoid getting hit as you simultaneously slap his arm to your right. That way his weapon and your head move away from each other, thus providing you with a slightly larger timing opportunity to slip in your counter.

On slippery grass, minimize movement by leaning away from the blow, while maintaining a stable stance, and then countering with an effective technique that uses only minimum movement.

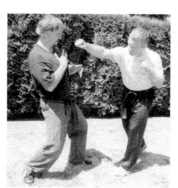 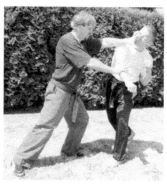

Practice 2 sets 10 reps evading, parrying and countering on both sides

Prepare for the worst

Despite your best efforts - maybe you slipped on the wet floor, he got in the first blow, or there was an explosion on the sun - you are suddenly thrashing around with your opponent trying your best not to go down. One of the many benefits of practicing on slippery surfaces is to gain experience knowing what it feels like when you start to lose your balance in a fight. Sometimes you can recover, but other times you can't, which is why they invented the word *splat!*

Recognizing the feeling that you are about to fall is crucial here, and it's best to get an understanding of it through your training. Learn of it in practice so that it doesn't take you by surprise in a real situation. Know that specific feeling of when you can no longer recover your balance and it's time to take the fight to the ground. While many instructors say you should never deliberately go down, sometimes it's just your best option when you are slipping and sliding and about to fall, anyway. This way you get to go down when *you* are ready and on *your* terms. To reiterate, it's not about dropping to the floor the moment there is trouble, no matter how skilled you are on the mat. However, when there is no more possibility of staying upright and you are flailing your arms around as if you were on a mosquito farm, you are susceptible to your attacker taking you down. When he does, he will do so to his advantage, to your disadvantage, and to your pain. You don't want him making the call, but rather you want to time the moment so that you go down when you are ready, and he gets the pain.

Minimize the impact of falling by using your breakfall skills. Better yet, since you don't want your opponent still standing when you are down, use him as the mat. Take him with you as you go down and twist as hard as you can so that you land on him. (It's okay to land with your pointy elbows and hard knees on his soft spots.) As soon as you both hit the deck, your priority is to get back up - not to grapple with him. You brought him down with you so that he wouldn't be in the strategically superior position of standing upright while you are down. Therefore, the moment you both land, your goal is to get back up so you can achieve that superior position. If you need to gouge his eyes or squeeze his groin to mush to do so, so be it. *Practice 1 to 2 sets of 10 takedowns*

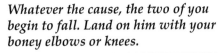

Whatever the cause, the two of you begin to fall. Land on him with your boney elbows or knees.

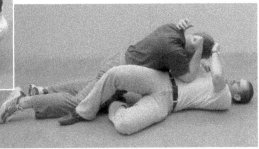

No matter what the combative situation - you are in a wonderfully wide-open field or you are in the dreaded narrow stairway on just-waxed linoleum - your goal is always to make a violent encounter a short one. If you have not practiced in environments that are cramped and slippery, you won't have a full understanding of your limitations or your capabilities. Not only will you be fighting a dangerous adversary, but you will be doing it for the first time in a dangerous, limiting space. However, when you have practiced and studied in these places, and then at some point you have to defend yourself in a similar environment in the real world, the dangerous adversary will still be a component, but at least the environment will be somewhat familiar to you. You will know how to adapt your timing to the specifics of the environment, and that will increase dramatically your odds of coming out on top.

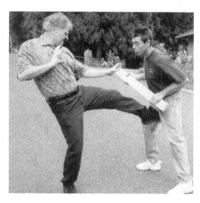

CHAPTER THREE

INTO THE MEAN STREETS

"I'm going to kill you," the man says. Well, that leaves little doubt as to what he wants to do. You don't know him, so how can you doubt his sincerity?

At the risk of stating the obvious: Timing is timing. It doesn't matter if the combat situation is occurring on the mats or on a rain-slick street. Timing concepts, principles, and certain techniques remain the same. The big difference in the street is the environment, the lack of a teacher to separate the combatants, the abundance of makeshift weapons, the concrete or asphalt "mat," and the ever present thought that a confrontation with a bully, a wrong look from a bar patron, a fight over a parking spot, a challenge to your manhood or womanhood, or a host of other issues, major or ridiculously absurd, could end up in a struggle for your life. In co-author Christensen's 29 years in law enforcement, he investigated hundreds of fights, big and small. Most were over the issues just listed, many ended with lost blood, some with serious injuries, a few ended in death.

All techniques and timing ideas regarding street confrontations discussed in this chapter have worked for our students (which include police officers and bouncers), fighters interviewed for this book, and for us. In other words, you aren't getting empty theory here. But before we get into the nuts and bolts, let's take a quick glance at three concerns about the person confronting you. The basic germ of these can be found in Sammy Franco's wonderful book *1001 Street Fighting Secrets* but have been modified to fit our needs here.

Don't bait the person into fighting

He might be woofing at you like a barnyard dog, but your antagonism, verbal or body language just might push him into getting physical. He has his ego and he might feel he has to save face. Besides, you should never underestimate a threat. He might look like a geek, complete with nine pens in a pocket protector and masking tape on his glasses, but that doesn't mean he can't put serious hurt on you, especially if he is armed with some kind of weapon. The more you indicate that you don't want to fight the better it looks later should the police get involved. More on this in a moment.

Leave him an escape route

Don't block his path. Just as you are always looking for a way to escape, consider that he might want to walk away, too. Purposely or inadvertently blocking his way just might force him to fight when he was only bluffing. Now, if he suddenly turns away from you in the direction of the exit, remain alert because he might not be going anywhere, but rather doing that old ploy where he pretends to go, then suddenly spins around with a sucker punch.

Determine his mental state

How is his demeanor? If he is intoxicated, high or mentally ill, understand that he is unpredictable and all your good verbal skills might not be penetrating his pickled brain. When he talks, listen to what he says, but more importantly, be alert and aware of his facial expressions, his tone of voice, and his actions. More on this in a moment.

Two techniques that almost always save your bacon

Will a fast backfist save you on the street? Yes. A powerful kick to the knee? Yup, that hurts. A finger in the eye, all the way up to the last knuckle? Of course. But there are two techniques more than any others that help to keep your nose centered on your face: alertness and awareness. While you can't always prevent volatile situations from happening, you can develop razor-sharp alertness and awareness so you can see trouble brewing before it gets to the physical stage. Without these two attributes, you are likely to find yourself *suddenly* in the mode of having to react to a threat. "Suddenly" has been italicized here to emphasize that the indicators were actually there all along, but you missed them. It's never good anytime a confrontation "suddenly" happens because, more times than not, it leads to poor performance and a lack of good timing moments for you – meaning, you get beat up.

Use a checklist

Here is what street specialist and author Marc MacYoung said in an interview about paying attention to what is going on.

"You need to develop a checklist. This checklist is made up of known danger signals, preparatory signs of an attack. These consist of things like someone walking up to you with one hand hidden, clenched fists, erratic eye movement, etc. You look for signs that indicate intent to harm you. Basically, you establish an external, verifiable standard that will tell you when it is time to move. Sometimes several items will be checked; sometimes just one signal will be so strong that it is enough to make the decision. Doing this list will take away much of the fear, because every time you checkmark an item, you become more certain of what will happen. If too many items get checked, you know it is time to act. It is no longer a guessing game of fear and emotions but a conscious decision based on facts. It boils down to being aware of your surroundings and what is going on."

MacYoung's thoughts also help prevent "brain clutter" when facing a person on the brink of fighting you. As the potential assailant moves in closer, calling you a colorful variety of obscene names, your brain works hard, sometimes struggles, to process the bombardment of all your thoughts: *Oh man is this guy big. He's getting closer to me. What did he just say? He's clenching his fists. What do I do? Man, his eyes look mean. A killer's eyes. Everyone is looking at me. Should I back up? No, I'll look chicken. Should I push him away? No, that will just make him madder. Is he going to hit me? Can he see my jaw trembling?*

However, when you have created a mental checklist of known danger signals and thought about them so they become embedded deeply into your mind, you create an environment, if you will, that is easier to function in. With the checklist in place, you take much of the confusion, concern and fear out of the moment, because the only thing you have to do is make little mental checks, and think about what you are going to do when the guy earns that final one on your list. All this takes place in the back of your mind, allowing you to focus all of your attention, strategy, and ultimately your physical action on what is happening in front of you.

The less confusion and brain clutter you have to deal with, the better able you are to seize the moment, to strike at an instant that is most effective. Think of brain clutter as baggage, extra baggage that you don't want to be dragging around when you need to be free and ready to respond when that window of opportunity opens.

Verbal Judo

Before we examine how and when to whack people with your fists, feet, and a beer bottle, let's first look at how to use certain verbal techniques to end a confrontation nonviolently. While these work much of the time, keep in mind that they don't work all the time. But they are worth mastering and implementing for the simple fact that if you can end a confrontation before it gets physical, you save yourself a lot of hassle. If he whacks you, you get hurt. If you hurt him, he might sue. Sure, he might not win, but it will cost you plenty in attorney fees to defend yourself over the average two-year period that a lawsuit takes. If you hurt him, you might get arrested, go to jail and have to take weekly showers with an ugly group of tattooed rapists, killers and dopers. It's definitely worth it to try some clever verbal techniques first. To be effective, you have to choose the right moment. It's all about timing, even with your words.

Verbal Judo, the book

Dr. George J. Thompson's book *Verbal Judo: The Gentle Art of Persuasion*, published by Quill, made the term "verbal judo" recognizable to hundreds of thousands who have read the book. Dr. Thompson is a karate black belt and a former English professor. He created and tested verbal judo while working as a police officer on an urban beat.

Whereas the art of karate involves two participants clashing head-on, the art of judo is about adapting, yielding, manipulating and using the aggressor's force against him. When two people stand toe-to-toe and scream at one another, they are using verbal karate. When one person uses the power of words, body language, facial expressions and even empathy to respond to an agitated person and redirect his negativity, that person is using verbal judo. More times than not, the end result is a deescalation of the volatile situation. Think of it as a gentle approach to taking control without creating additional stress, agitation, frustration, and physical conflict.

Say you are in a crowded public place maneuvering your way to the restroom when you bump a man who is holding a big cup of soda pop. He spins on you and barks, "Hey man, what's your problem?"

Clearly, this man isn't interest in your problems. He isn't expecting you to say, "Well, I'm starting to lose my hair and my cat keeps shredding my curtains." No, his words are a preface to a fight or at least an attempt to intimidate you. Don't fall prey to this.

Immediately assume an I-don't-want-to-fight stance, maintain a neutral facial expression (as opposed to sneering or rolling your eyes), and say, "I'm sorry, sir. My fault."

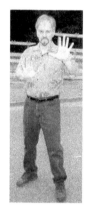

Sir? You should really say, sir? Yes, for the simple reason that it has power. Though you might think the man is a bicycle-seat sniffing loser, when you say "sir," there is a good chance it will melt him a little, or at least he will be taken back. He is expecting you to come back with something like, "What's *my* problem? What's *your* problem?" But instead you show him respect, almost as if raising him onto a pedestal. You aren't, of course, but don't tell him that.

Apologize politely

Your deescalation posture - open hands, relaxed body and calm face, what we call the I-don't-want-to-fight-stance - shows that you don't want a problem, though you are actually (and secretly) in a combat stance. Stand calmly, and move your open hands ever so slightly to affect a light stroking action. Psychologists say that this subtle movement has a calming effect on some people, but not everyone. Keep that last part in mind.

Assume the posture immediately when the guy says, "What's your problem?" and then follow with your, "I'm sorry, sir. My fault." The faster you respond, the more sincere you appear. Think *timing*.

This takes some people back. They cough, and go, "Well, okay. Be more careful." And the moment is over. Yes, you had to swallow a little ego, but you avoided a confrontation that might have escalated into a brawl. A couple hours later, you have forgotten about it and once again life is good.

Let him vent

But for some, your quick apology and "sir" won't be enough. These are jerks or the types who have to push the issue to impress their friends. Sadly, there are a lot of them out there. They are the ones who, after you apologize, ask challengingly, "You blind or something? This shirt cost 50 dollars and you're gonna pay for it. You must be a stupid and blind..." And on and on he prattles. If you try to explain further, he just talks louder.

The solution might be to let him vent. If he has a need to rattle on a little more, let him. Just nod and listen patiently. Nodding doesn't imply that you agree with him, but indicates only that you heard him. When he starts to wind down, apologize once more and move away. Take two or three steps backwards in your I-don't-want-to-fight posture to create space and to better watch him, then turn and walk away, glancing occasionally over your shoulder to ensure he isn't coming after you. Is this hard to do? You betcha. But if you can avoid a fight and all the related problems, it's worth it to swallow a little dignity and just feel satisfied in your mind that if you had wanted to you could have done a major rearranging of his facial features.

Try an insert

Let's say his words are such that you feel he isn't just venting, but he is working himself into an attack mode. The time is ripe to try what some psychologists call an "insert," one to three words that insert through his verbiage and into his mind like a sharp knife. Standing in your deescalation stance, you say, "Whoa!" Yes, whoa. It works on horses and it works on some people because of the implied command to stop. The man stops to see what you are going to do next. "Wait a sec" is another powerful insert. So is, "Listen." Both have an implied command to stop. Now, the person isn't going to stop for long, so it's a good idea to have something to follow with.

"Whoa. Let's talk about this, sir." You aren't telling him to shut up but suggesting that the two of you talk about the issue. There is no "What's *your* problem" back at him, but rather a phrase that means "let's you and I have a discussion." "Let's." Let us. Timing-wise it looks like this. The instant he challenges you:

• Assume an I-don-t-want-to-fight stance.

• Apologize.

That doesn't work and he begins to work himself into a state of agitation. Before he gets too worked up, you:

- Interrupt his verbal tirade by slicing into his mind with an inoffensive command for him to stop talking. "Whoa. Listen."

- He hesitates, and you initiate a conversation about the issue.

As he begins to lessen the intensity of his tirade, you:

- Follow with another apology.

- Maintain a relaxed body, neutral face, even voice tone, and an overall look of earnestness.

Can you see the timing involved in each phase? This works on lots of people, though it doesn't always work on the terribly drunk, terribly high, or terribly stupid. At least give it a shot and let other people hear you say the words and see your I-don-t-want-to-fight stance. If the man is simply brewing for a fight and nothing you say and do placates him, at least you created some witnesses in your behalf when the police come. "Officer," they will say. "That man (you) clearly didn't want to fight. He had his hands up and open and he asked the bully if they could talk about what happened. Heck, he (you) even apologized a couple of times. I heard him." This is good data for the police to know because it makes you look good.

If none of this works - and it works more times than not - and you have made a mental check on nearly every item on your checklist, start looking for the time and way to get away from him or, if there isn't one, start thinking how you are going to time your defense or offense.

Avoid fighting, avoid court

With few exceptions, your legal obligation is to avoid physical confrontation. If you have the option or opportunity to avoid using force in defense of yourself or another, you must avail yourself of that option rather than remaining and fighting. The myth that the one who threw the first punch is automatically the one at fault or is criminally culpable has been eroded to the point of non-existence. Self-defense is an exception to the rule -- but a narrow exception.

Self-defense is not simply fending off an attacker. It generally requires that there exist no other reasonable alternative available to end the confrontation. You tried to talk to the person and you looked for an "avenue of escape," a legal term meaning a way for you to get out of there. Standing and fighting is almost always looked upon with suspicion by district attorneys, judges and juries. If you don't have a way to escape and there is an imminent risk of serious physical injury to you or someone you are defending, you can use the *minimum* amount of force necessary to stop his attack and allow you to get away.

Know when it's time to get physical

"I'm going to kill you," the man says. Well, that leaves little doubt as to what he wants to do. You have to assume he has bad intentions based on the words he chose. In many jurisdictions, however, the law says that this type of threat is vague because the person threatening has not said how he is going to do it, nor is there an indication that he has the means or opportunity. Absent some other comment or action on his part indicating both a present intention and the ability to carry out the threat, you might not be justified in making a pre-emptive, or offensive counter-attack. Therefore, it would be in your best interest to try verbal judo techniques and find an avenue of escape, a way out of there.

Now, if he says, "I'm going to beat you to death with this pool stick," he has added a means to his threat, but only if he has hold of the stick or it's within his reach, that is, he has a means and an opportunity. If it's in the trunk of his car parked outside in the driveway, you can't jump him. But if there is one right there, and there is no way for you to escape, few district attorneys would charge you with a crime should you take an offensive action.

Here are the three elements needed before you can fight him. You need all three.

- **Threat** Has the aggressor said or done something that indicates an imminent threat to your safety or someone else's?

- **Opportunity** Does the aggressor have the opportunity to carry out the threat? Conversely, does the defender have a reasonable opportunity to escape or retreat, or otherwise avoid the confrontation?

- **Means** Does the aggressor have the means to carry out the threat by virtue of a weapon, his hands, feet, or the like.

When your alertness and awareness indicate that these criteria have been met, it's time to take a preemptive step. Let's look at a few techniques, based on precise timing, to neutralize the threat before he gets physical.

Hit the moment he threatens

If he is standing before you with a board in his hand, a scowl on his face and telling you he is going to beat you to death with it, attack him. Chances are he is expecting you to tremble, back up, or whimper. Instead, seize the moment when he is expecting fear from you, and slam him. Use whichever weapon of yours is closest to whichever target of his is closest. If your lead foot is close and he has his legs spread – hello! If you are in a I-don't-want-to-fight stance and your left arm is close to his face, palm him. In both of these cases or any others that you use, follow-up as needed with additional blows or flee if you have an avenue of escape. *Practice 1 to 2 sets of 10 reps of various scenarios*

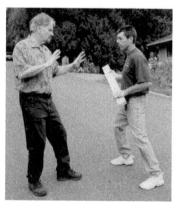 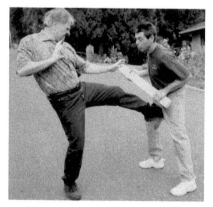

If the assailant says, "I'm going to beat you with this board," and you can't get away kick him in the groin.

Grab the moment he threatens

A technique that worked for Christensen when he worked as a policeman was to use his closest hand to grab the threatening person's closest shoulder and turn him. "Oh yeah, cop? You're not taking me, 'cause I'll kick your--" Christensen's closest hand would snap out and grab the subject's shoulder or upper arm, or the clothing over them, and jerk him around 180 degrees. Christensen would then dump the surprised person on his back, ram him into a wall, or apply an arm lock of some kind. More times than not it caught the subject completely off guard and, by the time he realized what was going on, Christensen had him under control. *Practice 1 to 2 sets of 10 reps of various scenarios*

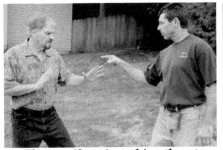
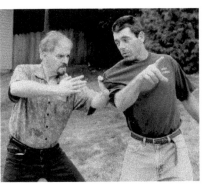

The assailant is making threats to hurt you. Grab his arm when it comes into your range.

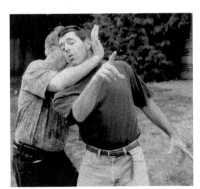
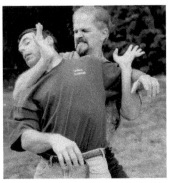

Move in for a head and arm restraint hold.

Say he makes a specific threat but the immediate timing moment for you to leap on him passes. Now you have to find another by watching for indicators that he is going to attack. As we discuss throughout the book, you want to move defensively or offensively the instant you detect an opportunity -- and you can as long as you have trained for it.

How to monitor

Most fighters watch their opponent's "triangle," that area formed by his shoulders and chin. Some watch their opponent's solar plexus, a few even look off to the side, finding that they can "see" the person better by not looking directly at him. Karate tournament great Dan Anderson has always watched his opponent's hands, as most police officers are taught. Some fighters argue that it's all about the eyes, because those windows to the soul give a person away every time. There is some truth to that, because an untrained fighter typically looks at what he is about to hit. If he intends to kick at your groin, he looks there first, or if he is going to grab the pool stick from the table, he gives it a quick glance. A trained fighter won't do that, unless he wants to fake you. He makes a quick look at your groin to distract you, and then punches you in the face.

Sammy Franco, in his book, *1001 Street Fighting Secrets*, writes, "Monitoring points are specific locations on your assailant's body that you should be focused on, including the throat triangle, shoulder region, hands, torso, and knees." He goes on to discuss that the monitoring point you choose ultimately depends on the distance you are from the threat, the type of confrontation it is, and whether the fight involves weapons or empty hands.

Christensen blends all of the above, with an emphasis on the triangle. Every movement - foot shuffle, leg chamber and arm motion - can be seen by watching the shoulders. The rest of the body is seen in the peripheral vision. If Christensen has some indication that the man is a puncher - the man has already punched someone out or has been drunkenly punching a wall - he monitors the triangle and the hands. If he thinks the man might be a kicker – he just kicked someone or is twitching his foot in preparation – Christensen monitors the man's shoulders and indirectly watches his feet in his peripheral vision.

Reacting to an indicator

Defensive response When you perceive an indicator, meaning you perceive the person's intention to do something bad to you, your ideal response is to explode offensively. Keyword: ideal. While it would be nice to be able to *always* beat a man to the punch, the reality is that there will be times when an attack comes so fast and furious, or a so-so fast punch catches you by surprise because you are having an off day, that you have to respond defensively. Block it or make a shield to take the blow on your arms, and then counter with any of the methods discussed in this book.

Offensive response   If you are having a good day and you perceive an indicator that the bully is going to attack, hit him first. If he draws his fist back to launch a big haymaker (what an amateur!), thrust your lead palm into his face, or kick him in the groin with your closest foot, or slam his knee with your instep. If he spreads his arms like a wrestler getting ready to charge, lunge and hit him first or sidestep and deliver a blow. Practice both responses in your training. If he lifts his leg to kick, leap in and jam it and then hit him. The key to success in executing an offensive response is to be alert for the indicator and, as a result of your training, have an immediate response to disrupt his attack and counter it. *Practice 1 to 2 sets of 10 reps of all of the scenarios*

Watch for suspicious hands Whether you focus on the triangle, or watch his upper chest, you still need to know where the threat's hands are at all times. If in his rage he begins clenching and unclenching his hands, be ready for an aggressive move from him. If he verbally threatens to rip your head off as he seethes and clenches his fist, *that* is the moment you want to make your move. He has told you *what* he is going to do and the clenching and unclenching of his hands implies *how* he is going to do it. It doesn't get much clearer than that. If you can't get away from him, attack him with your closest weapons.

People who carry weapons most often conceal them in the small of their backs, as well as in their waistbands at the front or at the side. So if a hand begins to make a deliberate move in that direction, be wary. If he threatens, "I'm going to cut you (or shoot you)," and you don't have an avenue of escape, explode on him without hesitation, and with extreme prejudice. *Practice 1 to 2 sets of 10 reps of various scenarios*

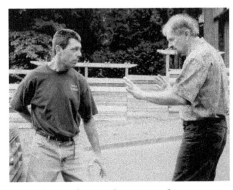 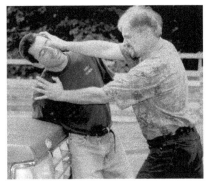

When he makes a threat to shoot or cut you and then reaches to an area where such weapons are typically concealed, jam his reaching arm and thumb his eye.

You are justified to move first in most jurisdictions if he made a verbal threat followed by a move with his hand to where you know from experience is a place where many people carry concealed weapons. (Your experience, by the way, can be from reading and being taught by professionals.) Furthermore, your fear was that if you waited to see the weapon, you wouldn't have had enough time to defend yourself.

The same response is justified should the man stick his hand under the flap of his jacket, as if reaching for a gun in a shoulder holster. This is a common ploy among gang members, street people and bank robbers. Does he really have a gun under his coat? Maybe. Maybe not. Are you willing to take the chance that he doesn't? What is your conviction based on that he doesn't? That he looks like a nice guy and is probably good to his mother? We're not telling you how to think here, but we do want you to know that naiveté from seeing the world through rose-tinted glasses can hurt you. On the other hand, we don't want you making false conclusions either and jumping a guy who is only scratching his chest. The poor guy has a rash and you punch him in the chops.

Look at the totality of the situation. Something sparked the confrontation with the man – you accidentally bumped him; you looked too long at his girlfriend; you owe him money; he is showing off for his buddies, or one of a thousand other situations – and now the two of you are looking at each other across five feet of space. The moment gets heated and he reaches under the flap of his jacket. "You're dead, *!@#! ^#," he growls.

For those people who still might think that that isn't enough for them to act offensively, we say, "Nice knowing you." To everyone else, we say, "Move NOW." You can:

- Lunge in and jam his reaching arm against his chest and palm-strike his face

- Jam his arm and throw him to the ground

- Jam his arm and push him against a wall

- Check his arm and run past that same side of him and out a door

Practice 1 to 2 sets of 10 reps on both sides of all options

There are many other responses you can make, but the point is that you have to move the instant his hand reaches. If you wait until he extracts a weapon, you might not have time to act, though you will have to make time to bleed. In most jurisdictions you are justified in attacking him given the situation: the *cause* of the confrontation, the man's *demeanor*, his *verbal threats*, and the overt action of *reaching under his jacket*.

A word on semantics

For purposes of clarity, we have been using the word "attack" to describe your actions when the subject makes a threatening move toward a weapon on his body. To be perfectly clear, your attack is in self-defense, a defensive move to save your bacon before the assailant presents a weapon.

Afterwards, when the authorities investigate the case and way down the road when the case go to court, it's paramount that you use the term "self-defense," not "attack." Don't say, "I attacked him when he reached behind him." Instead say, "Out of fear for my safety, I punched him to keep him from retrieving his weapon. I knew if I waited, I might be cut (or shot)."

Furthermore, don't let an attorney trick you into using the word attack. If you have to, interrupt him and say, "Excuse me. I didn't attack him. I defended myself from *his* attack, what I feared would be a deadly attack from him." And then look at the jury with big, frightened doe eyes.

The legality of you moving against a man who has yet to throw a punch is much clearer when he cocks his fist back, makes a verbal threat, and shuffles toward you. He is showing you a weapon (his fist) and he is sending you words that make his intention clear. You want to make a fast exit, but there is no place for you to escape. It's clear at this point that you have to use force.

His cocked right fist and his right side are angled back slightly, with his left hand fisted or, if he is untrained, opened and impotent at his side or near his front.

There are a number of responses you can make, and whichever you choose, you have to act the instant he draws his fist back. You can:

- Slam your closest foot into his groin.

- Lunge to his left side (away from his fist), grab his left shoulder and upper arm, and spin him around. Then do whatever you want to him.

- Lunge to his left side, check his left arm so he doesn't get frisky with it, and pummel him with your other hand.

No matter what you do, it has to be timed so that the assailant's fist is back and the same side of his body is turned slightly away. That gives you a beat of time to move in before he can rotate his body back and launch his punch.

Practice 1 to 2 sets of 10 reps on both sides of all scenarios.

Available weapons

Not only must you be alert and aware of the person's hands, body, verbal threats and demeanor, you must also be cognizant of potential weapons within his reach. If your confrontation is in the middle of an open, barren field, you have to worry only about getting struck with a handful of dirt. But if you are in a crowded bar, someone's home, alleyway or parking garage, you are surrounded by oodles of available objects that can turn a pushing confrontation into a potentially deadly one.

During co-author Christensen's police career, he was confronted with nail-studded sticks, 2x 4 boards, a coffee table leg with a two-inch protruding screw, wine bottles, a rifle, dogs, fruit, rocks, garbage cans, and a host of other items, none of which were brought to the confrontation by the people involved. All were picked up in the immediate vicinity, and used.

Weapons lying all about   Look around you right now. Whether you are riding on the subway or in an airplane, sitting in the bathroom or in your car, standing on the corner or in line at the movie, look at all the weapons within your reach. A briefcase, flower vase, rolled up magazine, hairbrush, telephone, cup of coffee, and this very book. All this stuff is available to you – and it's also available to someone angry at you. Always keep this thought in mind: though the person might not have brought a weapon to the fight, he could be armed in the blink of an eye should you fail to pay attention for a moment. The solution? Pay attention. Be alert and be aware.

Let's return to that bozo with the pool stick you bumped earlier. Whether it's his stick from home or one that belongs to the bar, he has it now. Is he threatening with it? Not at the moment, but it's in his hand so you have to factor that into the equation. You might say, "Hey, I'm sorry I bumped you. How about putting the stick down so we can talk about what happened?"

Some people say, "No problem, man. I don't need no stick to bust you up side the head." And the pool stick gets tossed down. Cool; one less thing to worry about. Others antagonists say, "You got a problem with my stick? You'd better because I'm going to shove it where the sun don't shine." While you would prefer that he doesn't do that, at least now you have information as to his intentions. So does everyone else within hearing, which is a good thing since there are now witnesses to his statement.

If he drops the stick, take the approach discussed earlier: Try some verbal judo. But if that doesn't work, choose the right moment to deal with him physically. If he threatens with the pool stick and keeps hold of it, your plan of action must include neutralizing it. He can poke with it, swing it like a baseball bat, or slash with it like Mushashi the great samurai swordsman. So as not to have to face any of those variations, you want to deal with him the instant *before* he puts the weapon into play.

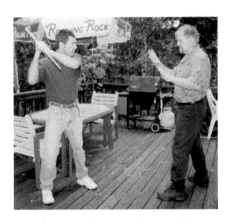 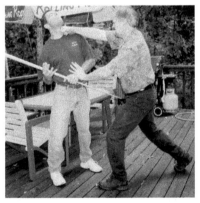

As long as the armed man is in an arguable nonthreatening posture, try to deescalate his anger with your words. But the instant he moves to cock the weapon, hit him hard.

Thus far, he has been standing in somewhat of a neutral stance. But just as he begins to chamber the pool stick, or as he changes his grip to a combat one, or changes his body position to one of aggression, or anything else that indicates clearly that he is going to attack, you want to explode into him. It's much easier to deal with him and the pool stick when you are in close, holding his weapon arm or jamming it against him, as opposed to standing back and trying to deal with a stick that is moving toward your head at 60 mph. *Practice 1 to 2 sets of 10 reps*

Let's change the scenario a tad and say that the guy you bumped is only watching the pool game and therefore isn't "armed" with a pool stick. However, he has been sipping from a beer bottle (his fifth, hence his attitude and courage) that sits on the edge of a table, within his reach. "You got a problem, punk?" he barks when you accidentally bump him. Here we go again. You try some verbal judo, but he is too drunk or stupid to be influenced. Somehow, you have gotten yourself backed into a corner so that there is no way for you to flee. You are stuck listening to him entertain his buddies by bullying and degrading you.

Always keep in mind that some people can get themselves worked up all by themselves, without the targets of their venom saying a word. Christensen has an 11-year-old dog, Chipps, and a six-month-old cat, Lexii. Chipps recognizes that Lexii is a mere child and stands stoically as the feline attacks him from below, above and from around corners. Sometimes the more Chipps just stands there taking it, the more Lexii gets herself worked up into an angry fit. When that happens, and it happens often, Christensen has to pull Lexii off before she starts to really rip into him. Well, some people are exactly the same way. Unfortunately, the guy you bumped is one of them.

As he rattles on talking about your mother, you note the bulging cords in his neck, his raised shoulders, his clenched teeth, and how his hands repeatedly open and close, all signs of a guy on the edge of exploding. You stand in your deescalation stance trying to get a word in edgeways, watching him for an aggressive move. Your I-don't-want-to-fight stance puts you in a good combat position, though it doesn't look like it, as he gets more and more agitated. He glances over at his beer bottle. You see the glance because you are alert and paying attention. When he snaps his hand over to retrieve it, you intercept his reach and deal with him offensively. A palm strike to his ear would be nice.

Practice 1 to 2 sets of 10 reps

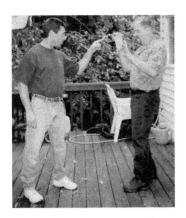
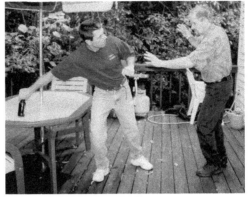

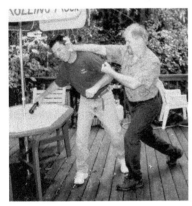

When he snaps his hand over to retrieve it, you intercept his reach and deal with him offensively.

Use minimum force

In self-defense, know that you can use only the minimum force necessary to prevent the assailant from hurting you. If you punch and kick him beyond what is necessary, you are at risk of going downtown with the police as well as being sued civilly by the very person who started the fight. Control yourself, control the situation, and avoid future legal problems.

Also, know that in some jurisdictions, if not most, should a guy pop you in the nose and then turn around and walk away, you don't have a right to go after him and crunch his nose. Since he turned around and is moving in the opposite direction, he is no longer a threat to you. Chasing him down and punching him would only be an act of revenge on your part, one that is frowned on by the law. (*Sigh*) Don't you long for the good ol' days?

No matter what your assailant is armed with or what he has available within reach, your best shot at neutralizing him and his weapon is your ability to seize the moment. The moment occurs because of an error on his part or because you suckered him in some fashion. Remember, it's a fleeting moment.

Look around you for weapons   It's critical to observe your environment for potential weapons. Consider everyday objects as lethal in the hands of someone wanting to do you harm. That cup of coffee could be thrown in your face; those scissors on that desk across the room could make a mess of your chest; those mechanic's tools could be used to stab or pummel. By taking a moment to see these objects as more than what they are intended for, that is, as things unhealthy for your flesh, you bring the many possibilities of their use to the forefront of your mind.

Co-author Christensen says he has investigated assaults in every conceivable environment. Many times victims would say something like, "I knew the frying pan was there on the counter, but I never thought she would smash me in the back of the head with it." Or, "All of a sudden he grabbed the garden shovel and whipped it into my legs. Who knew he would grab it?"

Well, the first person *should* have thought about being hit with that skillet, and the second person *should* have considered the shovel as a weapon. If they had thought about the possibility ahead of time, they might have taken measures to move away from the objects, or tried to maneuver the agitated person away from them. If such efforts failed to work, each could at least have been on guard for the possibility of these things being used. Then when the angry person reached for them, the other could have applied precise timing to neutralize the threat. However, preventative measures won't even be a thought if the potential weapons aren't considered a threat.

A nice side benefit of examining your environment is that you recognize various common objects as potential weapons that you can use, too. Just as you check out every restaurant, bar, carnival, and building lobby for potential threats when you first enter (you do, don't you?), you also want to give a quick look for weapons. Does this sound like paranoia? It could probably be argued that it's borderline, but know that a quick, nonchalant visual sweep of a new area takes about five seconds and, after a week or two of doing it every time you enter a place, it becomes automatic, an unconscious action. It's all about being prepared for a timing moment by being alert and aware of the surroundings.

Making a quick visual sweep of a new environment reduces or eliminates the chance of being caught off guard should the loud mouth you noticed when you first came in decide to toy with you. Instead of having to play catch up as to who he is and what he is about, you already have some idea. Also, your quick scan revealed where the doors are and where various objects are should he grab one or should you need to grab one.

When to use an environmental weapon

A bully has you backed against a corner, taunting you. He says he is going to kick your butt into the dirt and enjoy doing it. Since you subconsciously scanned your environment, you know there is a wooden chair about eight feet away, a wastepaper basket behind you, and a beer bottle on a table three feet to your right. This is all good information to have at the ready. But at the moment your plan is to use your karate techniques if the situation deteriorates to violence, and it's looking more and more like it's going that way.

"You really think you are leaving here with that pretty face, boy?" the guy snarls, straight out of B movie.

"Look, I'm sorry I offended you, sir," you say. "It was my fault. Let's talk about it as gentlemen." This is good verbal judo, but it's not working on this bozo because he came into the situation bent on hurting you. And because he is a stupid idiot. As noted before, there are a lot of these people out there, men and women.

"I'm going to cut that pretty face of yours," he sprays, his beer breath burning your eyes. "Cut it reeeeal good." With that he reaches with his left hand behind him, turning his body slightly to the left.

Perhaps you have heard the Latin expression *carpe diem*, meaning seize the day. Well, this guy is reaching for a blade and you don't have all day. You have only this moment, so you *carpe momento*: seize the moment. And you seize it NOW!

Thinking that because he is going for a weapon you should have one, too, you snatch the beer bottle from the low table with your right hand. Since he is twisting slightly to his left, you diagonal step to your left. Instead of taking the time to bring the bottle up and then back down on his head, you sweep it horizontally into his groin. Check his upper body with your left hand so that he doesn't spin around, and then use that bottle again, this time to smash against his closest kneecap, or his groin again if he isn't bent over too far. He drops in agony and you jump over him and flee. *Carpe momento.* It's good to know a little Latin.

Practice 1 to 2 sets of 10 reps on both sides.

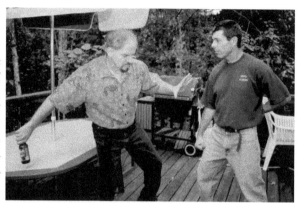

Your verbal judo fails and he reaches behind him for a weapon. You grab a bottle you noticed earlier, and whip it into his groin. To be sure he doesn't follow you out the door, whip another strike into his kneecap.

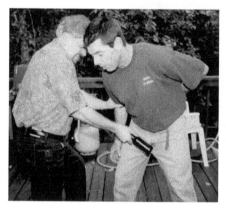
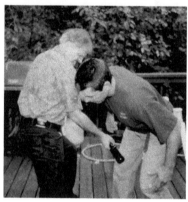

Think of an environmental weapon as a supplement to your martial arts techniques. Actually, hitting with a beer bottle or with a chair *is* a form of martial arts. If it helps, call it *beer bottle-do* and the *tao of chair*. Yes, you could have stepped diagonally left and whacked his groin with your palm and then round kicked his knee, but the beer bottle has a much harder striking surface. Yes, you could have probably pushed him back with a hard shove or an elbow smash, but if you push him over a chair that you have maneuvered him in front of, he lands with much greater impact. It's all about choices. But if you choose to use a weapon, you need to first be aware that weapons exist wherever you happen to be, and you need to pre-think how you would use them long before you ever get into a confrontation.

When sitting in your car

Let's look at one more scenario. Co-author Christensen used this numerous times as a police officer. Say you are sitting behind the wheel of your car at a red light, window down, elbow on the sill, oblivious that you have angered the motorist behind you in some fashion. Or maybe you do know you angered him, and you are trying to appear nonchalant while the light takes forever to change to green. In the side mirror, you see the guy scramble from his car and stomp angrily in your direction. Is that steam coming from his big nostrils? Hard to say, but he is carrying a board and you know he isn't a nice guy just wanting to build you a birdhouse. The name calling and threats make it pretty clear, too.

Strategically, sitting behind the wheel of your car isn't a good place to be. You can't kick and your punching and blocking ability is limited. Since the guy is a fast walker and you are having a slow thinking day, he is at your door before you can poke the lock or roll up the window. What was that Latin term? Oh yes, *carpe momento*. Given your vulnerable position behind the wheel, his rage, and the presence of a weapon, you are on solid ground legally, at least in most jurisdictions, to defend yourself. And what do you have readily available? Your door: a couple hundred pounds or more of steel and tin.

Stand next to any car door and you can see that if it were pushed against you, it would strike your midsection, upper thighs, knees and shins, depending on the contours of the particular door. When any one of these targets is struck, it usually knocks the recipient back. Sometimes the impact staggers him while causing the top half of his body to bend forward. A second hard thrust of the car door strikes the person's flailing hands, arms, chest, and even his head if he is bent over far enough. Such an impact buys you time to get out and flee, get the attacker under control or, if the light changes, drive off.

When Christensen worked Skid Row, a crowded, poverty stricken area, populated mostly with winos, drug users and criminals of every ilk, officers often parked their patrol cars at certain busy intersections as a deterrent and to keep an eye on the busy sidewalks. Any officer who worked the area for at least a few months could tell a story of a street person trying to punch him through the car window or hit him with a bottle. One fellow officer got his eyes gouged.

Christensen recalls several times when a belligerent person charged his police car door with thoughts of playing havoc with the co-author's face. "The car door was my friend, my partner," Christensen says. "As soon as the guy was within range of the door's arc, I'd release the door latch and give it a mighty push. Every time it smashed into the person's legs and chest and sent him yelping and stumbling backwards. Then we'd leap out and take the guy into custody."

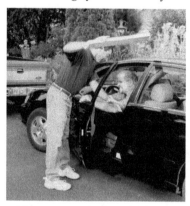 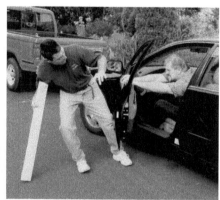

The moment he is within range, hit him so that top part of the door frame hits his face and the bottom section hits his legs. Hit him again as he falls away

Be familiar with your car door's arc. Analyze it so you understand exactly at what place a threatening person would have to be to get the full impact of the door. If you wait until he is too close, it won't hurt him or knock him back. Push it too soon, it misses him and bounces back closed, ruining your element of surprise. *Practice 1 to 2 sets of 10 reps with a partner.*

Free tip: After you have slammed it into an assailant, don't put your leg out too quickly. Christensen did that once and the bad guy shoved the door back and Christensen's leg got crunched. Hesitate for a second to see that he has been knocked back sufficiently (and to see if you need to whack him again).

If we could make this book a thousand pages longer, we could examine many more environmental scenarios, but even then we couldn't cover all the possibilities, as there are so many situations, places and people. Maybe you never frequent bars, but you spend your days in a computer lab. Or maybe you spend much of your day at a health club, or you work 24/7 on a farm. There are lots of possibilities for weapons in these environments and those of countless other lifestyles. Consider the possibility of a confrontation in them, the types of personalities who frequent these places, the potential for weapons, and how you would deal with them. Get detailed in your fantasizing and create moments when timing is critical, when you need to *carpe momento*, seize the moment.

Timing against big guys

One glance at the bruiser and you know that he shops at the Big N' Tall store. He is a foot taller than you, as big as a mountain range, and he has muscles everywhere, even in his hair. Making matters worse, he doesn't like your face and he is talking about moving your nose over there, and your chin a little farther to the right. You should have stayed in bed, but you didn't so now you have to deal with the gorilla. He is big, strong and mad, and your best hope is your ability to apply precise timing. First, using a good choice of words. Here is another Christensen technique, a maneuver from the street dance of cops and crooks that worked several times for him. The key is to insert a compliment when the guy appears on the brink of exploding. "You're a big guy, sir," Christensen would say, disguising his false sincerity. "You gotta weigh...what, two fifty? Looks like it's all muscle, too. What do you bench?"

This accomplished two things. First it stroked his ego. Big guys, especially iron pumpers straight out of prison, love to have their ego stroked because many of them, in their sad minds, feel that their size and muscular development make them superior. So when you feed that belief, they pause and they listen. It's a form of the insert that we discussed earlier, similar to "Whoa!" and "Wait a sec!" The guy wants you to tremble before him, but instead you compliment him. When this technique works, it makes the big guy quiet for a moment, partly out of surprise because your reaction isn't what he expected and partly out of wanting you to continue with the compliments. Sometimes you have to take it a step further.

"I really don't want to go toe-to-toe with you because you must out weigh me by a hundred pounds." Notice there is no real, overt admission of fear, nothing about how it would be a good fight, and there is never a return threat. There is just the recognition that the guy is big. Christensen says he would never say something like, "You know, you could pick me up and toss me out into traffic," since he wouldn't want to put any thoughts into the guy's head that weren't there before. The idea of the compliment is to punch through the guy's brain for a second to give him pause so that you can attempt some other verbal judo techniques. With some big guys, just the acknowledgement of their size is all they need. Then when you immediately follow with something like this, "There is no need to get physical. Let's just talk this out. Look, I'm sorry if I offended you in some way..." you regain some control of the situation by getting his focus off you and onto him. To make this work, you have to time it so that you insert it at the right moment, usually when it appears the guy is about to take the argument or confrontation into the violence arena.

Christensen says this worked like a charm - *but* - he is quick to point out that it didn't always work. When it didn't, it was time to put on some music: Olivia Newton John's classic, "Let's get physical."

Facts about big dudes

Big and strong might be significant or it might mean nothing at all. Martial arts author and teacher Bob Orlando says, "Strength alone, like brains, means nothing. It's knowing how to use your advantages and abilities that's important -- not simply having them." Martial arts instructor Frank Garza says that often the big guy doesn't have great speed and efficiency of movement but, he is quick to point, there are some big fighters who can move fast. He adds that many, though not all, fatigue quickly. If you can last with the big guy, his fatigue provides you with timing opportunities.

Big is also relative:

- If you weigh 250 at six feet four inches, a guy weighing 260 at six feet, five inches isn't that big a deal to you, unless you know for a fact that he just won a mixed martial arts, full-contact championship (and he beat his opponent to death with the guy's ripped-off arm).

- Even if he isn't a martial artist but you stand five feet, four inches, the guy appears to be a behemoth.

- Now, if he is just a mountain of blubber, never having lifted a single dumbbell or worked a physical job in his life, he isn't much of a threat at all if you weigh 250 at six feet, four.

- Even if you are five feet, four, the fat guy isn't nearly as intimidating, and even less so if you are a highly-trained fighter.

- If he is a blubbery 250 but he is a former state wrestling champ, your concern would be higher, no matter what your size, though probably greater if you were five feet, four.

- If he is a muscular 250, but a card-carrying wimp, your concern would be a little lower, though you would not want to lower your guard.

An example of a big wimp   One of Christensen's police partners investigated a spousal abuse call in which a Mr. Universe winner, a monstrous guy who had graced the cover of every bodybuilding magazine at least once, had beaten his wife. When the officer walked into their house, the big guy locked himself in the bathroom, crying like an infant and refusing to come out because he was afraid the police would, as he whimpered from behind the door, "put bruises on my body."

We could go on and on with more variables but let's just make it easy and say that the tattooed wonder towering over you is one big !$@$#. You have tried your verbal judo and it fell on deaf ears. So now it's time for Olivia to sing her song. Let's look at some timing options.

Against a good punch/kick fighter

Say your big guy looks confident as he assumes an upright, boxer-like stance. Maybe he isn't a trained martial artist, but you have seen him use his hands and feet in the past, and you know he is comfortable fighting at a distance with his long limbs. Understand that that is *his* fight, not yours. Use your footwork to stay out of range and to keep him turning left and right as he tries to follow you. When he throws a hand attack, evade or block and try to punch his attacking arm, aiming at vulnerable targets. Punch the fine bones on the back of his hand, the largest part of his upper forearm and his biceps. Then scoot out of range. If he kicks, try to evade his big legs, but if you have to block, counter with a solid punch above or to the side of his kneecap, or to the highly vulnerable peroneal nerve that runs down the outside of his thigh. If you feel he is off balance, zip in and strike a vital target – groin, support knee, throat and eyes – and then scoot out quickly.

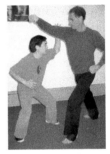
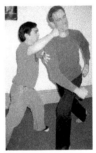

Keep in mind that since he has those cursed long arms and legs, he has more time to react to your moves and he takes comfort in that it takes you a tad longer to reach him. If you telegraph your intentions, be prepared to go, "Ouch, you broke my nose, big fella," and he will no doubt do it from outside of your range, but within his. Therefore, to play the game your way (actually, the street isn't a game), try to draw him to you. *Come on big boy...show mama what you got.* Then when he throws that big punch or kick, evade or block it, then follow as he retracts it and lay some business of your own on his vital targets. If he punches with his right hand, follow to that side, away from his other hand. When he kicks, follow it back and counter. It's amazing how well this works when you time it just right. *Practice 1 to 2 sets of 10 reps on both sides of attack defenses*

Against a good, but slow big guy Say that after a few seconds into the battle you find that the big guy is a good technician, skilled at a variety of techniques, and appears to be experienced. But Mother Nature cursed him with lots of slow-twitch muscles, or maybe he has plenty of fast-twitch but he is so darn big that he just can't move all that mass quickly. First, look up to the heavens and mouth a silent "Thank you," and then prepare to unleash your mighty fury on the guy.

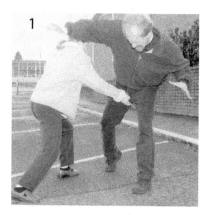

It's impossible for even the most skilled fighter to attack without leaving a large opening somewhere on his body. Since a big guy is, well, big, his openings are big, too, so much so that you could drive a Ford truck through them. This is good news. Now your strategy is to take advantage of his wide-open spaces with perfectly timed counters.

He throws a right punch at your face. Dip underneath it and slam a hard strike into his groin with your right hand, whip your left elbow into his ribs, strike his groin with your right again, and then scurry out of there. *Practice 1 to 2 sets of 10 reps on both sides.*

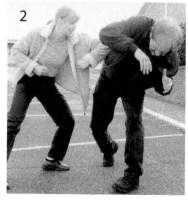

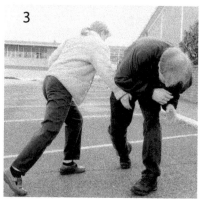

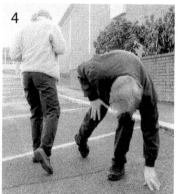

If he launches a straight kick, block the outside of his leg and scoot forward to counter with a strike to his face from the outside, or sidekick his support leg. Better yet, get behind him and have fun punching and kicking him before he turns around. If he launches a circular kick and you block it on the inside of his leg, slap the top of your foot into his groin, scoop kick, or sidekick his support leg.

Practice 1 to 2 sets of 10 reps on both sides.

Against a bad puncher   While there are many fast big guys, there are probably more who aren't, especially among the untrained. Should you get an untrained, slow guy, life is good, as long as you don't let him get a hold of you. An untrained, slow bully often tries to load up his Volkswagen-sized fist by drawing it waaaay back behind his shoulder, and then drawling in his best John Wayne voice, "Why I oughta..." Should you encounter one of these, pump your relatively little fist in the air, and go, "Yes!" then bash him. (Wait. You better bash him first.) Assuming you are unable to backpedal and escape, move in on him the instant he draws his fist back. You can do this in a variety of ways because his thought process, at least for a moment, is on his punch smashing you in the face. You can:

• Use your closest foot to slap upward into his groin.

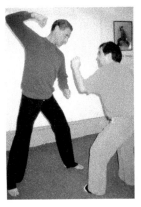 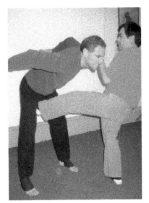

• If he is cocking, say, his right hand back, diagonal step to your right and round kick him in the closest available, vulnerable target.

• Lunge in and palm-check the shoulder of the punching hand and elbow him in the closest, available vulnerable target.

• Lunge in hard and fast and slam your forearm against his upper chest, throat or face.

Practice 1 to 2 sets of 10 reps on both sides of all attack defenses

No matter what technique you choose, you must time it to the drawing back of his fist. Since he could be faster than you think, shield your head with the arm that is on the same side as his chambering punch, while staying alert for a sneaky punch from his other hand. Don't waste time punching his chest as if it were a tournament match. You aren't going after points with the big guy; you want to wear and whither him down as a result of your carefully chosen punches and kicks to vital targets. Time this right, and victory shall be yours.

Against a bad kicker Say the guy has attempted a couple of kicks, making it perfectly clear that he is an untrained, awful kicker. He is like a lot of people who kick without knowing how: He ends up off balance and stumbling, and his drunkenness isn't helping him. Sweet!

He kicks again. You evade it easily and pause a half second to let him land and teeter on the brink of falling. Know that as he lands, his mind is on his balance, actually, the loss of his balance. That is when you seize the moment to counter punch him, kick him, or even grapple him in the direction he is stumbling.

Practice 1 to 2 sets of 10 reps on both sides.

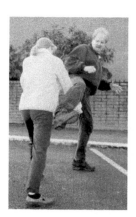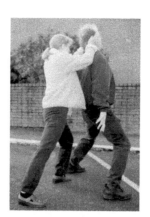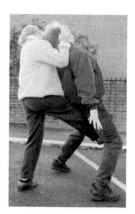

Block his sloppy kick off to the side. Scoot behind him to slap his ears and then shin kick his groin as you pull him off balance.

When the fight lasts longer than you hoped In a perfect world, you would use your savvy and awesome techniques to knock the big boy on his big bum. But life and fights don't always go the way you would like. Let's say that for whatever reason the fight is still going on two minutes after it began (most are over in a few seconds) because the guy is good at eating pain or he has been able to move just enough at the last second to diminish the effectiveness of your blows. Whatever the reason, the fight is still in progress and you are so glad you have been working on your aerobic fitness. What to do now?

You have been able to keep him at bay and you have been able to hit him a few times using good timing, but the blows have not had much effect. You are concerned that he is losing respect for your abilities, which could lead to greater aggression from him. Time to make a believer out of him. If you have landed a groin kick (which he shook off), throw a fake kick there to draw a reaction from him. He might have tolerated the last one, but he still didn't like getting kicked and will try to prevent another. When he drops his hands, slam a hard palm into the side of his neck. Next, throw a fake to the same place on his neck and, when he goes for the block, drive a Nike into his crotch. Should he drop his hand reflexively to his groin (though way too late) smack him in the neck again.

Understand that you aren't standing there toe-to-toe with the guy, because if you err, he will make mincemeat pie out of you. Stay moving. Scoot forward and back, diagonally left and right and sideways left and right. Each time you move into range, fake and follow with a hit, or just hit directly. Strive to impact vulnerable and sensitive targets, and use your footwork to confuse and frustrate him. Your objective is to gain his respect and possibly make him fearful of you. Once you have that, he is yours to play with and to finish off.

Free tip: Although there are exceptions, most big guys aren't terribly fast. This is an important consideration when determining the speed of your fakes. Bob Orlando says, "Greater size usually indicates slower speed (it simply takes more energy to move greater mass). Feinting or distraction work well as long as your response is not too quick. You want to capitalize on his reaction. Let it play out and don't pounce too soon."

If you throw a fast fake and he reacts to it slowly or not at all, do the next one more slowly. The same is true of drunks, but even more so. Co-author Christensen says that before he learned this, he would throw a fake at an intoxicated person or make some other distracting movement. Not only did the guy not react, he wouldn't even blink because the message took too long to process in the guy's pickled brain. Christensen learned to hold his fake out for a second or two to allow it to be recognized and then responded to. We don't recommend that you hold your fake for a one-thousand-one count with a sober big guy, but just long enough for him to respond.

When you don't know how he will fight   Most of the time in a street confrontation you won't know anything about the guy, other than he is as big your car and appears to be stronger than you. Don't underestimate him and don't apply any big-guy stereotypes: He is slow; he is dumb; he is a bully with nothing to back it up; he will back down when you call his bluff; and size doesn't matter. While stereotypes sometimes contain shades of truth, there are no absolutes. Always, and there are no exceptions, be aware and alert of everything the threat is saying and doing from the first second of your contact to several minutes after. Consider that your first impression and your stereotypes might be completely wrong. You might be thinking about using your super kicks to nail him from a distance, but then he throws a fast and beautifully executed kick at you. If you weigh 160 and you are a good kicker and he weighs 220 and he is a good kicker, you need to change your game plan right then and there because you don't want to fight his fight.

Don't let his size psyche you out. Yes he is big, his eyes burn with an insane intensity, he has a panther tattooed on the side of his neck, and there are lots of big chains draped all over his sleeveless, black leather jacket. While these are symbols of a tough guy, you aren't fighting his clothes, his eyes, or his tattoo. You must deal with his techniques and his strategy, just as you have many times in your training with other people. Clear your mind of the symbols and ready yourself for whatever he offers you: fist, kick or shove. Once he reveals his first move, and it might not be an offensive one, say, he drops his guard or looks to the side to wink at his buddies, unleash a mighty storm on him. Use any of the timing concepts we have been discussing to strike hard and fast at whatever available targets are hanging out there. It might be your only chance, so unleash a tornado of techniques on him, complete with thunder and lightning.

Taking the big guy down

While this book isn't about the technical aspects of grappling, let's look at timing as it relates to upsetting a big guy's balance so you can take him down using whatever technique you decide best fits the situation. The simple concept described here works on a lot of people. Note that we said "*a lot* of people," meaning, it doesn't work on everyone.

A few years ago, after Christensen had been studying grappling for about 20 years, he was feeling pretty good about his ability to "read" an opponent's balance, that is, to know through his senses where the person's balance was weak, and then apply a quick technique in that direction to take him down. Christensen's confidence was based on training with karate students and doing it for real on untrained combative people on the job as a police officer. Then one weekend he trained with a 30-year veteran of jujitsu, a martial artist who was expert at how to unbalance others and how not to let his opponent unbalance him.

"He was like trying to take down a building," Christensen recalls. "Starting from a clinch, and without the help of kicks and punches to weaken him first, I could barely budge him. I'd shift my weight, fake a pull or a push, but the guy was always a click ahead of me."

Fortunately, the average thug on the street doesn't have this skill, though he might have picked up some real-life experience that makes him more formidable than a less experienced street person. Still he is easier to deal with than a veteran jujitsu or aikido person. (Don't read into this to mean you don't have to respect the guy or be alert to his every move, because you do.) This is because unlike veteran grapplers, average fighters are careless with their balance, making them highly susceptible to taking a nosedive onto the concrete. Let's look at the simple concept of balance.

A quick lesson about balance Humans should be a tripod, meaning we should have a third support leg, like a camera tripod. We do just fine on two because our equilibrium continually works to keep us upright, although we are all somewhat weak in the direction of where that support leg would be if we had it. Stand up and assume any foot position you want and then look to see where that support leg would be on either side of you. That is the position where you are susceptible if someone gave you a little nudge in that direction. Lean your body over that spot, even a little, and you multiply your susceptibility. In other words, it won't take much of a push or pull to send you crashing to the earth.

The especially good news about this is that big guys, people with heavy upper bodies, are often more susceptible to being unbalanced when they are leaning away from their center. There are exceptions to this, especially with big guys who have been trained and can recover quickly from an unbalanced position, or can do nasty things even when off balance. Most, however, are vulnerable to being taken down when precise timing is combined with proper technique.

How to unbalance a big guy   There are two ways a big guy can become unbalanced. He inadvertently does it to himself: He slips, over reaches, or his attack puts him off balance. Maybe you did something to make it happen: You threw a fake, foot swept him, your block knocked him off balance, or you forced him to trip over something. No matter how he got to his unbalanced position, you need to move quickly to take advantage of his momentary weakness.

Say he throws a big arcing haymaker, which you lean away from, though you still feel its breeze on your face. Freeze frame: His big, missed right punch has left him with his right leg forward and his upper body leaning forward and a tad to your right. If you didn't take advantage of that brief moment and dump the big oaf, you are back to square one. Here are some options to do when you are having a good timing day.

- If his punching arm is across his body, grab his inner elbow and upper arm and yank him down in the direction he is leaning.

- Grab his hair, tuck your elbow and jerk him down in the direction he is leaning.

- Grab his hair with one hand and his shoulder with the other and yank him down in the direction he is leaning.

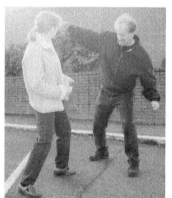
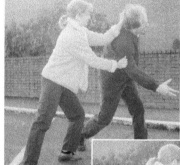

*The big guy swings drunkenly.
Let it pass, then move against his
unbalanced posture to grab his hair
and upper arm, and jerk him to his
knees. Run or finish him off.*

- Kick him in the groin or lower belly to keep him bent over and then grab whatever is available to pull him in the direction he is already leaning.

Practice 1 to 2 sets of 10 reps of various scenarios

There are many other techniques you can do so feel free to insert your favorite should you prefer it to any of the above. No matter what the technique, though, you have to apply it the instant you see the opportunity because, unlike in the last paragraph, there is no such thing as freeze frame. The moment is, well, momentary. Aikido instructor Stephan Stenudd says, "Make optimal use of the peak moment of the other one's attack: [Move at] the end of the strike." We agree and emphasize that this doesn't mean you react after his attack, at the very end of the timeline discussed earlier. Instead, begin evading as soon as you see his attack, and then counter at just the right moment at the end of his blow.

In the above scenario, the bully made the decision to swing and you took advantage of his awkwardness. You can also force some opponents to attack by bating them to punch at you. Say you are facing a man who is drunk, stupid or both, and you feel that he would strike at you should you be within range. Gutsy fighter that you are, you deliberately expose your chin. *Watch* him; your timing is critical here. Just as he prepares to launch his fist, step back so that he has to reach awkwardly toward you. Karate veteran Dan Anderson concurs: "Right as he begins to move, step back and overextend him." When he does, leap on him like a mouse on a 230-pound block of cheese, and take him down in the direction he is weakest.

You also need to move quickly when the big guy loses his balance backwards. Say he throws a kick and it causes him to lean back 20 degrees or more. Or maybe you threw a fake at his face and it surprised him to the extent that it momentarily shifted his weight backwards. Don't pause to congratulate yourself, but launch a second technique to knock him down in the direction he is vulnerable. Here are more:

- If his hands are flailing backwards, lunge forward and slam his chest with a powerful one- or two-hand shove. This works especially well when there is a chair, fireplug or curb behind him.

- Lunge in and execute a palm strike or palm push to his chin to knock him the rest of the way over.

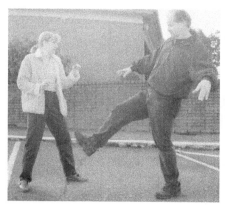
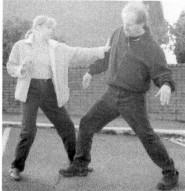

The big drunk kicks sloppily and lands off balance, his weight leaning back. Check his closest arm.

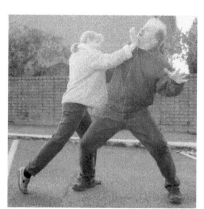
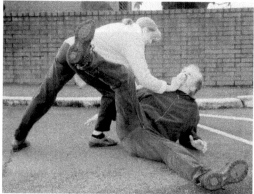

Palm his chin to drive him in the direction he isleaning for a takedown.

- Drive a powerful front kick into his midsection that delivers both impact and shove.

- Scoot in and execute a foot sweep, pulling it toward you so that he topples backwards.

Practice 1 to 2 sets of 10 reps on both sides of the various scenarios

To reiterate, the concept here is to nudge the big person in the direction he is already leaning. This works on fighters of any size, but it's particularly effective on tall, heavy guys because they have so much weight leaning off balance. When you attack him precisely at the right moment, he will go down with a big *Whump!* But be warned: Get there a half second too early or too late, you might end up as the big guy's toy. Success is all about pre-thinking what you would do in such situations and practicing hard on precise timing in your training.

Timing against a gun threat

Note: Volumes have been written on gun disarming. While we could easily write 200 pages on this life-and-death subject, most of it would be beyond the scope of this book's subject matter. Instead, we address a few basic timing issues for you to consider.

You know that cool fake kick where you start to front kick your opponent's groin, but then you roll your hip and change it to a roundhouse kick at his nose? And you know that neat-o jump thingy where you spring up in the air and backfist at the guy's head? Well, should you ever have the misfortune of having to face a person holding a gun on you, forget those things because they are a definite shortcut to the graveyard.

Here are some considerations you need to factor in when thinking about disarming someone holding a firearm on you.

You won't see the trigger pulled

It takes very little movement on the assailant's part to pull that trigger. It's not as if he were preparing to launch a roundhouse kick that involves lots of body leaning, shoulder movement, foot turning, and so on. To pull a trigger, he only has to move just one little body part ever so slightly. So slightly, that it's nearly imperceptible to your eye.

First things first

When thinking about gun disarming, too many martial artists think about what they are going to do to the guy: deliver an offensive blow, take him down, kick him in the head, and so on. While these are good things to do to a person who has threatened to kill you with a gun, there are a few other things you need to do *first*, such as getting your body out of the line of fire. If you don't do that, you might not get a chance to do all the other techniques.

Moving is all about when

Initially, it's not about how you move or what you do, it's about *when* you move. Timing. Your first objective is not to get shot. As co-author Christensen remembers, rubbing his shin, getting shot really hurts.

"Run, Forest. Run!"

If you are 10 feet from the gunman, consider turning and running. If it's clear by his threats and his demeanor that he is going to shoot you, what do you got to lose by trying to get away? Statistics show that the hit rate is low when someone shoots at a running person, but it's quite high when the person just stands in place (especially when he has his thumbs in his ears, wiggling his fingers, and going, "Neener, neener, neeeeener.) Don't bother zigzagging as you flee because safety experts say that it doesn't help. Just run as fast as a gazelle.

Read your gut feeling accurately

If you are standing 10 feet away and your gut tells you he is a little hesitant, consider advancing toward him as you try to deescalate him with your words. It's critical that you don't confuse gut feeling with denial. Your gut feeling that he won't shoot is based on his words, actions and mannerisms. Denial is based on wishful thinking and believing that nothing bad will ever happen to you. Advance on him only when the information you perceive indicates he isn't yet on the verge of pulling the trigger. Can this be a difficult call? Oh yes. (That is why you should never volunteer to be a gunman's hostage.)

When you think the moment is right – based on his words, demeanor (he isn't in a rage and his hand isn't shaking), his finger isn't on the trigger, and there have been no absolute threats to shoot – advance slowly with your hands up and open in an I-don't- want-to-fight stance, saying calmly and evenly: "Let's just talk. There's no need to hurt me. I'm not a threat to you. Please don't hurt me." And whatever else your gut tells you might work on this particular individual. Stop when you get within striking range of him. When the moment is right for you to attempt a disarm – he looks away briefly, his gun arm lowers, he looks confused, or he begins talking – go for the gun. If the moment doesn't feel right, keep talking or get him to talk, and watch for a timing opportunity. Here are a few. Practice 1 to 2 sets of 10 reps of various scenarios.

- He looks away ever so briefly

- He gestures with the gun as he talks, moving it away briefly from your body.

- He turns his body away from you.

- He slips or stumbles.

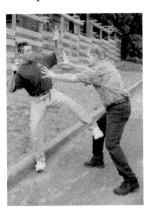

The instant he stumbles, you explode forward to secure the gun hand.

- He struggles to think about his words.

- He doesn't react to you gesturing with your hands when one or both of them come within in touch proximity of his weapon.

Here are a few considerations as to the technique you choose.

- The right technique for the job is determined by how and where he holds the weapon – one- or two-handed grip, at the front of your head, back of your head, stomach or your back-- and where your hands are at the moment -- down at your sides, up in the air, or behind your head.

- Since speed, as well as timing, is critical, you want your hands to take the shortest route to the weapon to move it aside as you twist your body away. The actions of moving your body out of the line of the bullet's trajectory and pushing the weapon aside, increases your chance dramatically of having a good rest of the day.

- If he holds the gun in his right hand, consider stepping to your left, away from his free hand, and knocking his gun arm across his body. From there you can jam his arm against him and apply whatever disarm fits the situation. Typically, more shooters are accurate when moving their weapon across their body (to the left for a right-handed shooter) than they are moving it to the outside (to the right for a right-handed shooter). This gives you a slight advantage since you are on the outside at his right.

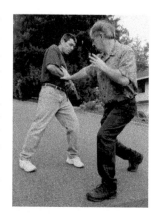

If he holds the gun in his right hand, consider stepping to your left, away from his free hand, and knocking his gun arm across his body

Timing against the blade

Note: Volumes have been written on knife defense. While we could easily write 200 pages on this life-and-death subject, most of it would be beyond the scope of this book's subject matter. Instead, we address a few basic timing issues for you to consider.

You have probably heard people say in training, "A knife fighter would never use a knife like that," or "A knife assailant would never attack with that technique." Nonsense. Knife assailants are made up of all kinds of people. In Christensen's 29 years of experience working around people with cutting devices, not one of them was a skilled, master, Filipino kali knife fighter. There were gangbangers with big folding knives, winos with shards of glass or broken wine bottles, prostitutes with hypodermic needles, and street people with hunting knives on their hips. None of them showed any particular skill with their weapons, although many of their victims got hurt, including police officers. Christensen says that his first week on the job he went to a family fight and found the wife sitting in an easy chair with a kitchen knife plunged into her throat. The assailant, her drunken husband, had not been trained with a knife, but how much training does such an attack require? At a different family fight, one that took place outside, the wife completely sliced her husband's ear off (it was eventually found under a car). She hadn't been trained, either.

When someone says that a person would never attack like that, ask where he got his information. Can he see the future? Never rule out anything in a fight. What this means is that when you train with knives, practice against all kinds of attacks: wild crazy flailing and clean sophisticated movements.

Say a street person is threatening you and you notice a knife sheath on his right hip. It's time to move the potential target - your body - but you have to decide in which direction. Since we aren't there to see all the variables that can affect your decision, here is some food for thought. You can:

- Sidestep to position yourself away from the weapon.

- Since it's arguably easier for him to slash with the blade across his body than it is to slash to the outside of his body, see if moving to the same side as the weapon is an option.

- Step in close to the weapon in preparation to jam the blade should he reach for it. The negative with this option is that you are close and can be punched with his other hand. No one said life would be easy.

- Look for something you can use for a weapon: chair, lamp, your belt, coat, and so on.

- If your avenue of escape is blocked, assume your deescalation stance and use your verbal judo as you maneuver yourself to where you can flee.

- Consider attacking. If he says he is going to stab you, know that his brain is either occupied with noting your reaction to his threat or with the process of reaching for his weapon. That is the moment you jam his arm and strike his eyes or throat.

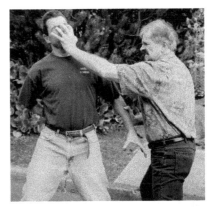

- The instant he reaches for the blade and you are close to that side of his body, jam his arm, gouge his eyes or punch his throat. If you are on the other side, out of reach, go for the eyes or throat. In either case, make your move the instant he moves. Don't wait for him to draw the knife.

If he says he has a blade and then reaches for it, believe him and attack.

Practice 1 to 2 sets of 10 reps.

Don't put a negative in your mind

When talking about knife defense, some instructors proclaim, "You're probably going to get cut."

What!? Why would they implant that in your mind? What if an algebra teacher said, "You are probably going to fail." Or the swimming coach said, "You are probably going to drown." What if as you sprint up stairs you tell yourself, "I'm going to fall and break my face on these cement steps."? Just as these things should never be said, you should never train in knife defense with a philosophy that you are going to get cut. Don't accept this negativity. Yes, it's a possibility, but keep that in a file in the back of your mind. You aren't in denial that it could happen. You just aren't entering the confrontation with I'M GOING TO GET CUT dancing in front of your eyes.

Fighting multiple opponents

All of the timing-related sport and self-defense techniques, principles and concepts discussed throughout this book also apply to dealing with multiple opponents, though it's necessary to reorganize your priorities a tad. Unlike in the movies, you won't scare off a mob by striking a fancy pose and letting out a high-pitched, panther-like Bruce Lee scream. You can try, but most likely everyone surrounding you is going to have a good laugh before they beat you into the sidewalk.

Veteran martial artists remember the early 1970s when the Hong Kong kung fu movies invaded our theaters. They depicted incredible fight scenes, especially ones where the hero pitted his skills against more attackers than could fit on the screen. If we are honest with ourselves, we must admit that as we watched the kung fu hero dispatch one villain after the other, we nodded a little to ourselves, and thought, "I can do that." Right, and barnyard chickens are good at playing the accordion.

The truth, however, is that outside the magic of the theater and into the harsh ugliness of the street, gamblers in Las Vegas would put their money on the attackers, not the lone martial arts expert. And more times than not, the bettors would collect because odds are that the martial arts expert is going to receive some serious injury, maybe get killed. This is because the lone defender not only has to contend with overwhelming firepower, but also the brutal nature of what is called "mob mentality." Like a half dozen shark fighting over one desperate swimmer, a mob can quickly become one mind as their "thinking" turns into a feeding frenzy, one of rib-kicking feet and blood curdling screams. Often the beating frenzy continues long after the point where a single attacker would back off.

When Christensen worked street gangs, he investigated many incidents of gangs encircling and attacking one, sometimes two victims. Several cases involved 40 or more gangbangers on one victim. In one case the victim was an elderly woman. His first case involved a pack of racist skinheads attacking a black man. One of the attackers was armed with a baseball bat and, at one point, stood over the fallen man and brought the bat down on his skull over and over, like a mad woodsman with an axe. So badly was the man's skull crushed that the medical examiner said it was impossible to conduct the usual autopsy procedure. We tell this story not to be morbid, but to point out the potential for a crazed mob mentality.

Are we being too doom-and-gloom when it comes to multiple attackers? Maybe. Although we are a couple of guys who view the martial arts with positive enthusiasm, and we provide you with some concepts here that will give you an edge when faced with more than one assailant, we also want to be perfectly honest and clear: There are absolutely no guarantees when fighting multiple opponents, as the odds are definitely against you.

Before we discuss some ideas, let's look at a few realities about group attacks. The realities are the exact opposite of all the myths about fighting multiple opponents, most of which have been shaped through movies. Always keep in mind that the movies are *reel*, not real. Here is the real truth.

- The attackers probably won't give you time to prepare for them. Most likely they will push you into a defensive mode quickly, forcing you into an OODA loop (see Chapter One) to slow your response or even make it impossible for you to respond.

- Your opponents won't line up single file and square off with you one at a time, face-to-face. Most likely they will act like a pack of hyenas, first circling and then moving in to blindside you. Some will taunt and curse you, while others will be silent, hang back, and wait for you to commit to one attacker so they can hit you from behind. Sometimes those are the most dangerous.

- They won't throw just one attack, which you easily evade and counter with perfect roundhouse kicks to the head. Most likely their punches and kicks will rain on you like a violent storm. Group attacks are chaotic in nature, and as such it can be hard to maintain a general overview of the situation when you are getting hit all over your body.

- If you aren't alert and aware of your surroundings, a group of attackers can have you boxed in and surrounded before you can mutter to yourself, "I should've gone to church more often." They are all about dominating, not about being fair.

- Assume there are weapons. The lower-IQ thugs tend to display theirs before using them, while the smarter and more experienced ones keep theirs hidden before bringing them into the scenario.

All the above unpleasantries are why you should never taunt a dozen street thugs. The only foolproof timing technique against group attacks is not to be where they are. But since you can't live like a hermit, there are specific measures you can do to avoid potentially violent groups and situations. Amazingly, there are some people who don't want to hear about them.

Case in point: When Christensen worked street gangs, he gave many safety presentations to neighborhood organizations. Whenever he would tell the gathering to cross the street should they see a group of obvious gangbangers hanging around the corner ahead of them, there was always one person who would stand up and proclaim that there was no way he would cross the street. "It's my neighborhood, and I have a right to walk down that street." Even after Christensen pointed out that crossing would add no more than two minutes to their journey and they would arrive at their destination unscathed, some people still insisted that they would not take the extra step.

Being sensible is being smart

Are you a coward if you take an extra step to avoid a potential problem? No, but you are being smart. Is a person brave if he wades into the middle of a problem? No. He is being stupid. If you see or sense a problem ahead, take a couple extra minutes out of your day to go around it, thus avoiding a potential situation that could very well have long-lasting effects on your body and your psyche. Bruce Lee called it "The art of fighting without fighting."

You pull onto the lot of a fast food joint and see a cluster of guys slouching around, flashing hand signs, wearing gang attire and glaring into your window. Think timing: "Okay, it's time to go somewhere else."

Awareness

If you walk around all day lost in thought, bumping into parking meters and other people, you aren't likely to perceive trouble when it comes into your space. Christensen says that many victims of muggings, assaults, attempt murder, and robbery would claim that the suspect came out of nowhere. Sorry, but that is impossible. The suspects were there all along, but the victims didn't see them until it was too late. Look ahead to see that unsavory character hanging around the next street corner. Look behind you every minute or so, to see those two guys behind you, trying hard to appear uninterested in you. Be alert to see those three men walking towards you and then separate, two to one side of the sidewalk and one to the other.

These are early (or late) warning signs of an impending group attack. Your awareness of them is a key factor in not only avoiding them but also dealing with them once it's too late to get away. It's difficult if not impossible to apply strategic timing in a defensive response if your head has been in the clouds and you don't know the threat even exists until it's in your face. Stay alert and aware to give yourself an opportunity to avoid a situation or, if you are unable to take an avoidance measure, at least give yourself an extra moment or two to seek a window of opportunity.

Types of groups

Let's break multiple attacks into two types: planned and unplanned, though there is some overlap. While it might be difficult under the stress of the actual situation to determine which case you are unfortunate enough to be in, it's helpful if you can figure it out so you can better strategize your defense.

Planned group attacks:

- A group of gangbangers are out cruising to do a robbery and there you are at the counter of the Freeze Delight buying your self a chocolate cone. Bad timing to go off your diet.

- That gal you have been dating for three weeks informs you that she is married and that her hubby, the bench press champ, and his weightlifting pals are out looking for you to have a "talk" about it.

- Several so-called wannabe street thugs are roaming the streets looking to beat someone up to establish their reputation. It's at that exact moment that you round the corner walking your little white poodle with the jeweled collar.

Whatever the case, the group is ready to use violence and each member is committed to a specific course of action. Some are more committed than others but in general terms, the cohesion is high and extremely dangerous. They have a specific objective and the desire to achieve it. This means it will be harder to break up or intimidate the group by overpowering one of them in front of the others, an often recommended course of action against a mob of less committed members. This driven group just might view your effort to do that as incentive to attack you with even greater rage. Their combined, albeit varied intensity, means they will fight more as a team than a group that hadn't gone out with a specific objective of hurting someone. Since every member is ready to fight, they typically move toward the intended target all at the same time. That makes any timing efforts by you extraordinarily difficult to carry out.

It's hit the fan　　Let's say you are cornered, your avenue of escape blocked. If your first thought is, "What a great opportunity to show off my jump spinning back kick," shake your head rapidly and make that idea go away. This spooky moment is about knowing which solid, basic techniques to use at the precise moment. It's about using reliable, meat-and-potato techniques and concepts to help you get home -- alive. Meat and what...?

Meat-and-potato techniques are those that require minor commitment of your bodyweight, can be done at high speed, and yield good results. Typically these include backfists, eye rakes, jabs and, if space and footing allows, snap kicks to the groin, moves executed quickly and with little risk of loosing your balance. To increase their effectiveness in this specific situation, target the eyes first. A quick finger swipe in an eye leaves even the toughest fighter wishing there was a referee to give an eight-count. At the very least, he is disoriented for a few seconds, freeing you to deal with the next opponent. The less time it takes to stop one attacker, the less chance the others have of getting you.

Get outta there　　Besides thinking about technique, timing and wanting to be elsewhere, you also want to be open for an available "hole" in the group so you can make a run for it. Think of them as a fence: They have you surrounded and locked in. You have to find a gate in the fence, or climb over it, or smash your way through it. Consider this scenario:

You are cornered and surrounded by three street punks. Fake to your left and then blast through the guy to your right. You aren't going to rat-atat-tat him with punches and kicks, but rather blast through him like a linebacker. But what if you weigh 130 pounds, about the same as a real linebacker's leg? Then blast into him as you simultaneously ram your fingers into his eyes (check out co-author Christensen's video *Vital Targets: A Street Savvy Guide to Targeting the Eyes, Ears, Nose and Throat*).

Do this right and add a dash of luck, the thugs will react to your fake to the left by moving in that direction. Then when you abruptly reverse directions, it confuses the guy on your right just enough to provide you with a small window of opportunity to get past him before he realizes your devious plan. If he is leaning a little toward your fake, your blast through should catch him off balance, maybe even knock him down. If he is particularly large or you are relatively small, stir your fingers in his eye sockets as if stirring a drink.

The whole idea is to escape without going toe-to-toe with the three attackers.

When you can't escape   If escaping isn't possible, the next option is to destroy the will of the group. This means you work to take away their desire to fight back and ultimately their commitment to their peers. Your success depends on the strength of their will and commitment, and the effectiveness of your techniques. If their will and commitment are stronger than your techniques... well, it was nice knowing you and thanks for buying this book.

Okay, we aren't going to leave you hanging. Here is a timing trick that can help.

Think of mobility as your best friend, and not moving as a way to get a fast ride in an ambulance. You must become a whirlwind of pokes to eyes, backfists to noses, and elbows to throats. When one guy lowers his arms to tackle you, gouge his eyes, and when he grabs his face and screams, seize the opportunity to ram your fist into the next guy's Adam's apple. Each time you cause damage, consider that window closed, and immediately look for another opening, or look for a chance to create one.

String them up   A common strategy for fighting multiple opponents is to "string them up," meaning you maneuver in such a way that your attackers form a column of sorts, so you can deal with just one at a time. This formation is usually short lived, as the group catches on and spreads out again. But it's good while it lasts because it's awkward for the attackers who have to move around the guy in front to get at you, which provides an extra second or two for you to deal with the immediate one. In essence, this means that you, for at least a moment, aren't fighting a group but rather several individuals, one at a time. In theory, this is a simple concept, but under the stress of a real situation it's difficult to pull off since your attackers seldom cooperate.

Training, of course, gives you an edge and a degree of experience at manipulating multiple opponents. One way to practice is to recruit a few classmates to act as the angry mob so you can work on positioning, footwork and timing. Get them to surround you in as many variations as you can devise, including ways that others are convinced would never happen. Then tell them to attack. As one training buddy steps close, rake your fingers across his face as you sidestep to move away from the other attackers. Now he is between you and the others. Good job, you just successfully "strung them up," but that doesn't mean the end of the training session. Your buddies keep on coming, as you continue to fight and maneuver them so you have to deal with only one at a time.

A progressive drill   At first, ask your training partners to take turns attacking you. Begin by defending against the first attacker with quick and efficient debilitating blows, all the while moving away. Don't hold your ground and hit, but *move* and hit. Then the entire group freezes so that you can orient yourself as to where you are and where the remaining attackers are. Use the same strategy and procedure with the next attacker: He attacks, you defend with debilitating blows while moving away, and then everyone freezes so you can study the scene. Once you get comfortable with this phase, you are ready for the next one in which the group attacks at will: all at once, one at a time, three at a time, whatever. There is no stopping and orienting yourself. Practice for however long it takes in each phase.

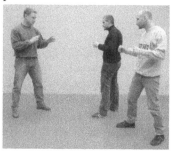
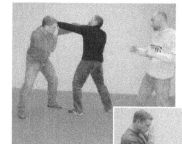

Face your partners. Parry and use a quick counter and step away to line them up. Grab his front kick and kick his groin

The drill teaches you how to combine your techniques with good positioning and precise timing. Move too soon to string them up and you run into another attacker, or several of them. Move too late and you risk not getting away from the next attacker or attackers.

Unplanned group attacks:

- You bump into a guy at a party and spill your drink on his shirt. He is drunk, angry and wants to make you pay, as do several of his buddies eagerly encircling you.

- You are in a bar chatting with a lady when her boyfriend, who has been shooting pool, sees you. In a jealous rage, he stomps in your direction with several of his buddies in tow, all salivating for blood.

- You pull into a 7-11 and accidentally bump your car door into the car next to yours. "Hey $@%!*," the driver shouts. It's then that you notice there are four other guys in the car, all wearing black bandannas, all with eye-piercing stares, and all getting out of the car.

Because of the unplanned nature of these incidents, there is a greater possibility that your verbal deescalation skills will work. Strive to calm them before they can build enough mental momentum to start swinging. Apologize, offer to buy them a drink, back away towards the exit, do whatever is necessary to avoid the fight. This isn't being cowardly, but about being smart enough to realize that you alone against two, three or more attackers is a no-win scenario. Should the group not back down or leave you an escape route, it's time to stop talking and prepare to rumble. But always, your main goal is to get away as quickly as you can.

Once the fight begins with the unplanned group you follow the same guidelines just discussed in "Planned group attack."

Planned and unplanned group attacks

The most striking difference between planned and unplanned group attacks is the lower level of commitment by the group that didn't plan, though that doesn't make them any less dangerous. Because there is no planning involved, there is usually not enough time for group members to get psyched and to mentally prepare. Still, some people can switch from quietly drinking a beer to ripping your head off in the blink of an eye. Others, though, need longer to get "pumped" to commit violence.

Types of attackers in both

Let's examine the typical categories of opponents in both planned and unplanned group attacks. Don't think of these as definitions set in stone because there are some types that overlap. Also know that under stress, it's not always easy to determine types.

- Depending on the size of the group, there are usually two along for the ride. They aren't really interested in fighting you, but they are enjoying the show and waiting until others do most of the work so they can jump in and kick you in the head a few times after you are down. These guys aren't the most dangerous, but they still pose a threat since they increase the total number of opponents you have to deal with.

- The bigger threat is usually the "mouth" of the group. He is the one cursing, swearing and hyping himself into a frenzy. The mouth or mouths, as sometimes there is more than one, tend to be the more experienced in the group and therefore the harder to deal with. Know that they can easily distract you from what the rest of the group is doing.

- You also need to pay attention to what the "silent fighter" is doing, too. This can be difficult because the guy is, well, silent and unassuming. But know that he is likely positioning himself to blindside you once he gets the signal from the mouthy one. Or he might decide to do it on his own. Though he begins silently, once he does move he typically charges in with great enthusiasm.

Here are a few timing tricks that have worked in these categories.

- Here is a great concept taught by self-defense expert, Marc "Animal" MacYoung, one that works best against the unplanned group. When the window of opportunity presents itself, attack the mouthy one and throw him into the silent fighter. This takes care of two of the most dangerous people, and can damage the fighting spirit of even experienced groups. At the very least, it can offer you a second or two when they hesitate, a timing moment in which you can bolt for the door and not stop to wave goodbye.

- A bouncer friend of Demeere's once faced three guys at a carnival, one mouthy and two silent. The bouncer waited until the mouth was in mid-sentence (mid-curse, actually) and grabbed him by the hair, yanking him sideways. This created a nice opening and a timing moment for a hard sidekick right into the first silent guy's midsection, who up to that point had been there only to enjoy the show. Oh, he could still see the show, but from the vantage point of being curled up on the floor, trying to breathe. The bouncer then choked out the mouthy one, while using him as a shield against the second silent fighter. The choke hold took 10 seconds to take effect, at which point the second one decided wisely that he would rather get out of there than face a guy who just dropped two of his buddies.

- As a self-defense instructor walked home one night, he passed a man who was sitting on a fence. Right after he passed, the man scooted off and began following, setting off alarms in the instructor's suspicious mind, even more so when he noticed another man sitting on a wall ahead of him. To test the situation, the instructor crossed the street to the unpaved, gravel side of the road and, sure enough, the man behind him crossed as did the man to his front. The self-defense instructor knew he was being set up for what is called a "pincer" move, where a street criminal from the front sets up the victim, as the other assailant jumps him from behind. It works because most people see the one to the front, but not the other. They figure it out only after they get clonked on the back of the head, and wake up with a headache and without a wallet.

  The instructor listened carefully to the man's footsteps in the gravel to his rear, and when he could hear them directly behind him, he spun and blocked the man's reaching arm. Without pause, the instructor slapped a chokehold on him, reached over his head with his other hand, and hooked his fingers in the man's eye sockets. With an insane expression and using his best Jack Nicholson voice, the instructor asked the other man, "Wanna go bowling?" Then shaking the first attacker's head for him, he added, "I've got *my* ball." The front man, armed with a pipe, circled him once, then wisely changed his mind and fled into the night. The instructor slammed a hard hammerfist into the choked man's sternum, dropped him to the ground, and then continued to walk home.

- Royce Gracie of the Gracie family Brazilian jujitsu fighters teaches that you might be able to make the leader fight you by himself. You say something like, "If you want to fight, let's make it just you and me, one-on-one. Or maybe you need help to fight me?" This attacks the leader's machismo since he isn't likely to say he needs help. It's even possible that his friends will encourage him to fight. Timing wise, don't wait until the entire group is chomping at the bit to get you. The moment you realize your verbal skills aren't working, that is when you challenge the leader.

Fighting multiple opponents is every martial artist's fantasy and every martial artist's nightmare. The fantasy is in seeing ourselves dispatch a horde of attackers with grace and coolness, without even raising a sweat. The nightmare kicks in when we stop to realize that the chance of winning such an encounter is poor to real poor. And our chance of getting hurt badly is good to real good. However, defending ourselves, at least to a point where we can escape, is possible when using one or more of the many timing strategies discussed in this section. Here are those timing moments all together as they apply to multiple opponents.

- The instant you see a group of suspicious people ahead of you, cross the street or take a different route to your destination.

- Be alert and aware of your environment to increase your reaction time and to see a window of opportunity before you are surrounded.

- Being able to determine quickly if the attackers planned the moment or just suddenly came to it is helpful when formulating a quick plan and taking advantage of a timing moment.

- Solid, basic techniques are usually best when seizing a moment of opportunity.

- Quick strikes to vulnerable targets generally work best when timing moments are short lived.

- Think of the attackers as a fence, so that when the moment is right you can make your escape by charging through or over it.

- Use body faking to create an avenue of escape.

- Stay mobile to keep from getting hit and to find more timing opportunities to act offensively.

- Try to "string up" the attackers to deal with them one at a time.

- If the group appears unplanned, try to verbally deescalate them before they get riled up.

- Consider taking out the mouthy one first.

- Look for a timing moment to take out the mouthy one along with the silent one.

- If there is one mouthy guy, challenge him to fight you by himself. Make the challenge before others in the group get psyched to beat you up.

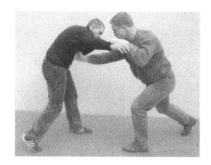

CHAPTER FOUR

IT WORKS IN A TOURNAMENT, BUT

WILL IT WORK IN THE STREET?

...your inability to adapt a tournament technique to the street doesn't make it worthless for self-defense.

Although the question of whether a particular sport fighting technique is applicable in the street is asked so often in training circles that it's now a boring cliché, it's still a good question, an important one. While many tournament fighters could give a hoot whether their stuff works against a street killer just as long as they win a plastic trophy, other sport fighters assume that their techniques will save their bacon. Then there are those martial artists who train solely for the street and ridicule sport fighters as living with false assumptions. Ooooh the controversy!

Well, your esteemed authors have taken it upon themselves to settle the debate once and for all. So, will sport techniques, concepts and principles work in a dark, damp alleyway where a prison-muscled, pitbull-tattooed, stringy-haired, low-IQed, tank-top wearing, Camel-cigarette-smokin' thug wants to eat you for a snack? The answer is...

It depends.

It isn't that we are chicken to take a side on the issue, but it really does depend on a lot of factors. It wouldn't be right, nor would it be safe to make an absolute declaration to one side of the debate or the other. We do believe that making blanket statements -- one-size-fits-all -- is dangerous. (Yes, we know that was a blanket statement.)

Some schools are sports oriented and others are slanted more toward self-defense. Which schools in our experience produce the better fighters? Again, it depends. There is a police officer in co-author Demeere's muay Thai gym who competes at the international level. He is strong, highly skilled and trains totally for sport: full contact, but still sport. Yet he is able to easily handle himself when police work requires that he use force, and it's his sports muay Thai techniques that he uses. Because of his extreme training regimen -- training until he drops, receiving and delivering full-contact punches, knee strikes and kicks -- he has well-prepared himself for the stress and intensity of the average street scuffle.

On the other hand, Demeere once trained with a highly skilled Silat player from a self-defense oriented school, a fighter who had collected hundreds of techniques and could deliver them with great speed. He was good but also cocky and aggressive when sparring with Demeere. When he refused to lighten his impact to vital targets, Demeere decided to play his game and hit back just as hard. Naturally, the game escalated quickly (Demeere holds no claims to having a high IQ), until the Silat player started flinching and choking up. He could dish it out well enough, but he couldn't take it because he wasn't used to getting hit, as was the aforementioned muay Thai fighter.

In the article *Facing Multiple Attackers? Styles, Attributes and Strategies for Successful Self-defense* written by author and martial artist Brad Parker (posted on www.defendu.com), he says, "I witnessed a highly-proficient Tae Kwon Do stylist knock down five opponents in a parking lot using classical TKD techniques. Three of the five opponents were dropped with head kicks! Many would say that these are impractical for self-defense, but they obviously worked well for this guy in this situation!"

Bottom line? It depends on the individual as to how effective he is in a real fight.

Always keep in mind that the art and skill of perfect timing isn't limited only to the question of when and where to hit, but also which weapon to use. As we will see in a moment, sometimes a head kick *is* the best technique for the open window. Christensen once executed a jump front kick that brought down a resisting subject after the man had just picked up Christensen's partner, a six-foot-two, 200-pound officer, and slammed him onto the sidewalk. As Christensen ran through a pounding rain to help his partner he saw a four-foot wide patch of wet grass between him and the assailant. Christensen said there was barely a conscious thought of doing a jump before he leaped through the air, flew over the slippery grass, and planted his size 11 right in the big guy's chest.

Many street oriented teachers say to never fake in the street, as is so often done in competition. Well, maybe a fake is the only thing that will expose a timing moment. Maybe a snapping backfist – a technique often ridiculed as ineffective in a street encounter – just might do the trick to snap the adversary's head back a little so you can slam a kick into his groin.

Are some point-fighting techniques weak? Yes. Should you not use a weak one though it's the best technique when that window opens? Of course you should use it. The old song that there are no referees in the street is exactly why you should use it. In a tournament, the head ref stops the fight after a weak technique lands to see if the judges want to award it a point. In the street, that technique can be used to "get through the window" and then, since there isn't an annoying ref to stop the clash, you can finish the adversary with more powerful techniques.

> *Don't rule out anything in the street.*

"That would never happen on the street"

Here is a typical blanket statement heard everywhere from taekwondo schools, to police defensive tactics classes, to kung fu halls, to women's rape prevention seminars. "An attacker will never (insert technique of your choice) in the street," says the instructor. Sometimes it's a student who makes this proclamation. Do you ever wonder how these people know this? Have they seen every fight, every mugging and every rape? Have they seen every method there is to attack or to resist a grappling hold. If not, then how can they make this blanket statement? Could it be that in their ignorance, or in their attempt to sound important or knowledgeable, that they are assuming and then stating their assumptions as fact?

It's like those so-called knife "experts" who say that a knife assailant would never cut you in such-and-such a way. Oh really? Says who? As discussed earlier, co-author Christensen investigated many cuttings as a police officer and never -- *never* -- was the attacker a trained knife fighter. The victims were attacked with overhead strikes straight out of a slasher movie, wild, drunken swinging motions, uppercut motions, the whole gambit. But never were any of the victims attacked with clean, efficient, highly-trained moves.

This doesn't mean that people don't get attacked and killed with clean moves, because it happens. In the horror that is war, there are warriors whose job is to take out sentries, usually with a brutal and well-trained knife slash to the throat. Or in countries and cultures where carrying *and* using knives is part of every day life, you are more likely to face people more adept at wielding a blade. However, for the vast majority of people in most civilized countries, this is rarely the case. The average American or European gangbanger doesn't spend three hours each day doing knife drills to ensure he gets the angles of attack right. He simply relies on a simple slash or thrust.

Few real fights are typical

Over the years Christensen patrolled the asphalt jungle, he either came upon in progress or investigated afterwards a variety of weird fights: a man who beat several other men with his artificial leg; he witnessed a man place another man's head over the edge of a dumpster and then slam the lid on his face; he rolled up on parents fighting over a baby, the father pulling on the infant's arms, the mother pulling on it's legs; he investigated a man who kicked a long-handled comb up another man's nostril; he saw x-rays of a convict's head after another con had rammed an unsharpened pencil through his ear canal and into his brain; he rolled up on two drunks exchanging face punches inside a car enveloped in flames, and who fought Christensen after he pulled them to safety; and there was a fellow officer who fought a man armed with a 12-foot bullwhip. Never say to Christensen, "An attacker would never do that in a real fight."

Never rule out any possibility. Never make blanket statements about what an assailant might or might not do, and never rule out what you might or might not do. The only blanket statement that you should live by is that you should never make blanket statements and never rule out anything.

"Sport fighting techniques will get you hurt on the street"

Oh yeah? Says who? Is there a guy in a white lab coat with a clipboard analyzing *every* street confrontation and making notations? Does he have a column for "Sport techniques" where he checks the "Didn't work" box? If there isn't such a guy, then how can the speaker make such a claim?

The fact is, he can't or, more accurately, he shouldn't. Even if he is a high-ranking martial artist, he can only make assumptions, albeit educated ones. Such as:

- "Fancy tournament techniques are risky on the street. Stick with solid basics."

- "Point fighters are used to tagging their opponent's and then scooting away."

- "There are no referees on the street and there are no timeouts."

- "Tournament fighters are used to pulling their blows and might do so on the street."

- "Only people with street experience do well in a street fight."

- "To survive in the street, you must become an animal."

We will comment on these statements in a moment.

As a martial artist you probably have had non-martial artists tell you about a karate guy or tournament fighter they know who got beat up in a bar. While there is always a possibility of this happening, after hearing it for the umpteenth time, it begins to take on the flavor of an urban legend. Ever notice that "the guy" never has a name, and that no one knows where it happened or knows where the guy is now? We aren't saying that it's never happened, but rather to take such comments with a grain of salt. Maybe even challenge the speaker. "Oh really. Who was it? Where did it happen? What were the circumstances? Was he taken by surprise? Was he outnumbered?" Nine times out of 10 you are going to hear "I don't know" in answer to every question.

Before we get to the subject of timing as it relates to sport vs. street, allow us to rant just a little more and comment briefly on each of the aforementioned bullets.

- "Fancy tournament techniques are risky on the street. Stick with solid basics."

  o This is true to some degree. While it's best to use less risky techniques that aren't about pretty but all about effective, there are people who can make tournament techniques work. Of course it helps if the adversary isn't a good fighter.

- "Point fighters are used to tagging their opponent's and then scooting away."

o While it's true that an explosive barrage of techniques might be the thing to do to finish off an assailant, there are many fights where only one technique is needed. Have you seen the video shown on those home video television programs of the karate tournament champ who interrupts a man abusing his girlfriend in the street? The footage, captured by a rooftop-mounted video camera, shows the karate man yell at the abuser who is on the far side of the street. After the man throws his girlfriend in his backseat, he charges across the lanes toward the karate champ, who waits casually until the man is in range, and then knocks him cold with a single backfist to the head.

In Vietnam, Christensen hit a Marine in the chest with a classic tournament reverse punch that sent the man's heart into fibrillation. It was touch and go for a while as to whether the man would survive. He did.

- "There are no referees on the street and there are no timeouts."

o There is a risk that the tournament fighter will develop a conscious or unconscious sense of safety knowing that there is someone to keep control and order in the pretend fight, and this sense can carry over to the street. There is less chance of this happening when the tournament fighter spends time training for and thinking about real fighting. That said, during our competitive years, we didn't train for or think extensively about the street, and the fact that there was never a ref present during our street confrontations was never an issue.

- "Tournament fighters are used to pulling their blows and will do so in the street."

o The argument here is that how you train is how you fight for real. So, if you train to pull your punches in practice and in the heat of competition, you will in a real fight, too. Sounds like a reasonable assertion, but it hasn't been our experience, or the experience of any of our students. It might be because when sparring and working drills we hit using medium contact, and we spend a lot of time hitting the heavy bag, hand-held pads, and other training aids to get a feel for hitting full force.

- "Only people with street experience do well in a street fight."

o Everyone has to have a first time. Does everyone lose the first time out? No. While having been in a street confrontation might give one a sense of the stress, adrenaline pump, and fear that accompanies a street clash, much of this is present, to a lesser degree or maybe more, in competition. All things considered, the trained fighter, even one without street experience, has an edge.

   Experience is only of value if you learn from it. A guy who gets jumped and beaten into the sidewalk has "street experience." It wasn't a good experience for him, but it was an experience. Even if he analyzed what happened, looked at all sides of the experience, he ends up knowing a lot about only that one experience. Christensen once used a wrist technique (sankyo) on a guy armed with a knife. Christensen says he didn't plan on using that particular technique, but it just happened when the window opened. Does that make him a knife fighter? He says no. He thought a lot about how he executed the move – how he stood, how he maneuvered the guy, what he said to him, how he cranked on that wrist – but his "street experience against a knife is limited to only that one, small incident.

- To survive in the street, you must become an animal.

o Why? You will just get arrested, sued and then go to jail. Your techniques might be named after animals, but your mind-set must be calm, strategic and calculated, just as it is in competition. Christensen got into a lot of resist arrest situations and all-out fights in his job as a police officer, but never once did he fight like an animal.

Sport techniques for the street

Okay, we are done ranting; back to the subject of timing. Let's look at a few techniques that are typically sport oriented and see how they can work in the street, particularly when applying precise timing.

Lead-leg roundhouse angle kick: Many fighters think that this kick is ineffective because it lacks power compared to a rear-leg one. These are people who probably don't have a powerful lead-leg kick of their own, or have never been nailed with a solid one.

Since there are lots of variables from one kicker to the next – speed, power, and accuracy – let's say, for purposes of discussion, that you have an average roundhouse. That is either a compliment or an insult to you, but let's make it average since an average one to the groin hurts most people, or at least makes them walk funny for a while. There are lots of ways to time the execution of this kick. Let's look at how to do it simultaneously with your block.

A street thug has been insulting and trying to intimidate you when suddenly he pops a jab at your face. In one motion, you snap your head back, swat his fist aside, pop your angle round kick into his groin, and return your foot quickly to the ground. In the event he has cast iron, uh, you know, follow with additional techniques. Here are two key elements to using the kick in the street.

- Don't pose with it after impact. Return it to the floor and nail him again in the same spot or scoot out of range.

- Know that groin kicks don't always have an immediate effect. Sometimes it can take a minute or more before that oh-so-special hurt comes calling. This is all the more reason why you need to follow up with additional blows, back away, or take an avenue of escape to get away from him. Christensen once caught a knee in the groin while scuffling with a wanted man in the lobby of the police precinct. The fight went on for another five or six minutes before the man was handcuffed. It took another four minutes to walk him to the back of the precinct and lodge him into a holding cell. It was then that that special pain hit Christensen like the proverbial ton of bricks, bringing with it nausea and ache. It took almost 10 minutes to get there, but when it arrived it literally stopped him in his tracks.

Something to think about A common trick in point fighting tournaments is for a fighter to try to get his opponent penalized by faking injury from his accidental groin kick. As the "injured" fighter makes a big production of rolling about on the mat, clutching his groin, and crying for his mother, the referee calls a foul and the crowd turns against the other fighter for playing unfairly. After the kicker gets disqualified a couple of times for this, he becomes hesitant to use groin kicks in competition, a hesitancy that can overlap to the street. To overcome this, he must train specifically for groin kicks in self-defense situations so that they become an instinctual weapon in his repertoire.

Drawing a punch

There is a strong debate among street oriented martial artists as to whether it's a good idea to deliberately expose a target to draw the adversary into hitting it, or more accurately, hitting at it. It works in tournaments and can be made to work in a real confrontation. Is it risky? You betcha. But does it open windows of opportunity for you? For sure. It does require self-knowledge that you have courage, speed and skill to carry it out, and it's also helpful if you have some knowledge of your opponent: he is drunk, he is a slow-moving bully, or he is just downright dumb. Here is how it works.

Stand in your fighting stance or in the I-don't want-to-fight stance, left leg forward. During the course of the confrontation, lower your left hand so that there is a clear shot to your chin. Your opponent spots the opening and launches a right cross or jab at your jaw. Since this was your plan all along, you either move your head out of the way, or snap a hand up to swat the attack off course, and then counter with the quickest technique for the job, say, a palm thrust to his face with the same hand that blocked.

Drawing is similar to faking except you don't make an overt action, like throwing a fake backfist. Instead, you simply open a path with the intention of drawing your opponent's technique. It's important that you practice with a live partner to see how much you need to expose, which defense is fastest, and which counter is fastest. Keep in mind that while you might be hoping for a right cross, he might jab at your chin with his left. Explore this possibility to see if you need to change anything.

Not everyone is fast enough and skillful enough to be able to draw an attack. Know yourself, know the risk, and train hard on it.

Practice 1 to 2 sets of 10 reps on both sides.

Drawing his body   In the last technique, you try to draw the adversary into punching you in the opening of your choice. This time you draw him into moving toward you so you can hit him using his forward momentum against him. Good tournament fighters use this as a surprise to catch the opponent off guard. In the street, it's used to add power and ultimately pain to your attack by creating a head-on collision between your outgoing force and his incoming force. It sounds great on paper and it is in reality, but it's not always easy to do. Doing it right is what superb timing is all about.

Have you ever watched two pro boxers or two upper-echelon full-contact martial artists punch and kick at each other only to have the knockout blows swoosh through the air without connecting? That is an example of missed timing, especially incorrect gauging of the right time to hit when the opponent comes in or when he moves away. So, if the professionals have trouble hitting at the right moment in the ring, will the rest of us have even more trouble landing a blow against a street thug, especially when trying to time our kick or punch to land as the guy advances? Our definitive answer is...maybe, maybe not. (Yes, that is another wishy-washy answer.)

It all depends on the skill of your adversary. There are some exceptional back alley fighters out there who have never had a boxing lesson or a "buy one month, get second month free" karate lesson, but still they have developed incredible skill from their experience in the streets or in prison. But, and this is a really big but, they more than likely don't have the skill of a highly-trained professional, or at least the experience of having gone hundreds and hundreds of rounds in training and in scheduled fights dealing with umpteen timing moments. See why our answer was so wishy-washy? That said, if we were forced to go out on a limb, we would say that as a trained martial artist, you will have an easier time implementing good timing on the street than you will against another martial artist of equal skill. Yes, yes, we know there are exceptions, but more times than not, it will be easier to apply a timing moment against Bruno, the local bully.

Let's use the same drawing technique you just used in, "Drawing a punch," except this time drop your lead arm when you are positioned just a little beyond his arm's reach. This greater distance forces him to lunge forward to hit your opening, which creates the forward momentum that you want from him. When he falls for the bait, backhand block with your lead hand as you did before, but instead of palming his face with the same hand, use your rear hand to drive a hip-twisting, rear-leg driving reverse punch into his solar plexus. Hitting as you did before with that lead palm causes some good pain when the adversary is standing still, and more pain when he is moving toward you. But when you step in with a rear-hand punch with good body mechanics to meet his forward momentum, he suffers from even greater collision power.

Practice 1 to 2 sets of 10 reps on both sides.

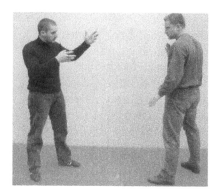
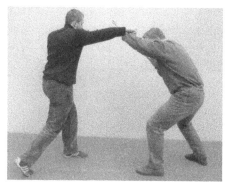

Drop your lead hand to draw your opponent's right cross so you can drive a hard punch into his solar plexus as he moves forward.

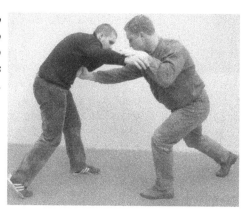

"Come here, big boy" Here is one more body-drawing technique, a goofy one that works in tournaments and in the street fights because of how it manipulates the brain - some brains, not all. You and your opponent are squared off in your stances. If you were in your fighting stance, fists raised and ready to go at it, you would move back in the usual course of moving about. If you were in the I-don't-want-to-fight stance, open hands up, you would move back as if trying to avoid the confrontation. Manipulating your opponent's brain comes into play when you make a subtle "come here" gesture with the fingers of one hand, or both hands. Amazingly, many people see the gesturing fingers and move toward them. But you must be subtle with the gesture - a couple little wiggles with your finger tips, not your entire arm as if you were trying to be seen by someone at the far end of a football field - so that witnesses can't say later that you were baiting the guy. The trick is actually funny when it works, except when someone plays it on you.

Say you are in a confrontation in the street and you have your hands up in a deescalation stance. Your gut tells you it's about to get physical, so you step back three, four steps, as if you were afraid, though you subtly gesture for the bully to come toward you. When he moves, you stop abruptly and lunge into him with a lead-leg front kick or, if you have time, the more powerful rear-leg front kick.

Practice 1 to 2 sets of 10 reps on both sides.

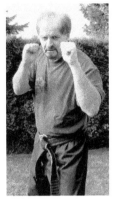
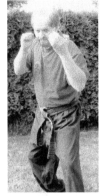
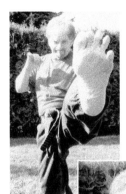

This is what your opponent sees. He sees your on-guard stance and then sees you move back. The subtle drawing of your gesture compels him to step forward, and right into your foot, or your punch.

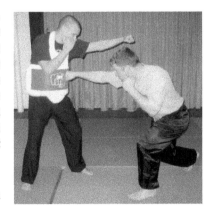

Padded partner To train for timing, get your workout partner to wear a chest protector while you drill on punching and kicking as you move into his advancing force. Punch too soon, and your fist hits only air. Do it too late and you just might tweak your wrist. Keep working until you educate your eye to just the right distance.

Practice 1 to 2 sets of 10 reps on both sides.

Swinging heavy bag This old standard works great to simulate an advancing person. Push the bag away and work on a variety of techniques with which to meet it head on.

Practice as many reps on both sides as you like.

Punching the body

If you have seen many point karate tournaments, you have seen body punches earn points that wouldn't have stopped an advancing kitten. Still, these weak techniques get raised flags and the winner goes home convinced he has killer punches because the judges reinforced his beliefs by awarding him points. Back when point karate first began, points were awarded for blows that would stop or seriously hurt the fighter if they hadn't been pulled. Today, it seems that points are awarded for any blow that lands on the upper body, no matter how light.

Some people argue that punches to the body aren't that effective, anyway. Well, this is true when it comes to the many body punches that earn points in tournaments, but we have been hit with good body shots over the years, the kind that wobble the legs, churn the gut, and make breathing a near impossibility. We have also seen other fighters, including boxers, go down for the count with a well-timed and well-targeted body punch. Let's examine some ways, using timing and target selection, that help turn a weak body punch into one that leaves a street thug sucking for air, and going, "Mommy?... (*gasp*).. I want my mommy...(*gasp*)."

Hit him just as he begins to inhale Speaking of gasping, here is a way to really make your adversary gasp for precious air. It requires impeccable timing and good speed, but the results are worth the effort. The trick is to drive a hard blow into his belly as he breathes in. Make sure it's *in*. His breathing is especially easy to see when he is panting like an old workhorse, maybe from your last clash. He sucks in air, blows it out, sucks it in, blows it out, begins to suck it in – *Fumpff!* your fist sinks out of sight in his soft belly. Even if he has a six-pack of ab muscles showing, they still have to relax for a moment when he breathes in.

Practice 1 to 2 sets of 10 reps on both sides.

If you are still at the stage where the street bully is cursing you but you know in your gut it's about to turn physical, and you have no avenue of escape, hit him as he ends his sentence and starts to inhale. He shouts, "You *!*&!, I'm gonna tear off your head and spit down your neck." (He begins to inhale) *Ku-wump!* Your big ol' motorcycle boot slams into his abdomen.

Now, don't focus too hard on this concept because you will just clutter your mind with anticipation and miss many other opportunities. Just keep it in mind for when that window opens.

Good body targets Old West Lawman Wyatt Earp once said, "Fast is fine, but accuracy is everything." We agree, but we also believe fast *and* accurate is a good thing, too. Combined, they make for tremendous, debilitating body shots. Here are a few targets to hit fast, hard and accurately. Be sure to step back afterwards so your adversary has an unobstructed place to crumple.

The liver: Your opponent's liver is right under the right side of his rib cage. You can drive in some serious agony by hitting with a left hook with your fist turned halfway between vertical and palm up. Shift your weight to your left leg and lean your body over it a little. Hit with speed and with your weight behind the blow. Think in terms of "digging" in deeply with your fist, then angling up a little on a diagonal path toward his opposite shoulder. Speed, power and digging all create a moment of pure pain for the recipient, just before his legs turn to Jell-O and he drops to his knees.

Here is a classic timing moment to slip in a punch to the liver. Your opponent is in a right-leg forward stance and pops a right jab at your face. You can either slip his punch to your left, or backhand block it with your right hand, as you step to your left a little. Dip to your left as you lower your left fist and then crank your waist hard to your right as you drive your fist up and into his liver.

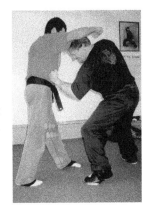

Practice 1 to 2 sets of 10 reps on both sides.

The solar plexus Many boxers consider the two best knockout points to be the chin and the solar plexus, the latter being the nerve center of the abdomen. Located at the top of your stomach and just below your pectorals, a hard blow to the solar plexus short-circuits the nervous system, often paralyzing the lower limbs. Hit yourself there a couple of times to get a sense of its vulnerability. Hit lightly! Sorry, we should have said that first. This area can be condition to a limited degree, though a blow there still hurts. Your average street bully has made his solar plexus even more vulnerable by routinely eating excess calories and bloating himself with too much beer. The solar plexus is most vulnerable to an upward-angled blow: an upward knee strike, a rising front kick, and an uppercut punch.

Here is a great timing moment. Say the bully throws a wild haymaker punch that not only misses, but also causes him to stumble forward off balance. His solar plexus is exposed and he has some forward momentum for you to use against him. Drive a knee hard and deep into his solar plexus.

Practice 1 to 2 sets of 10 reps on both sides.

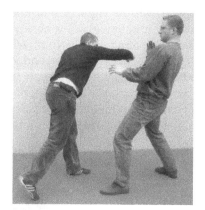 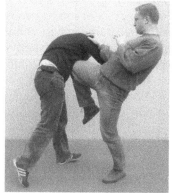

When your opponent's haymaker throws him off balance, ram your knee into his ribs or solar plexus.

Floating ribs: The floating ribs are those lower two ribs located at the front and sides of the body. Since they don't enjoy the same support as the other ribs, they are more susceptible to being broken. Even if they survive a powerful punch or kick, the muscles to which the floating ribs are attached can be strained or even ripped. This can really hurt, but the good news is that it only hurts when you breathe. It's also possible for a broken rib to punch through the recipient's lungs, heart and liver. If you are responsible for such a severe injury and the law finds that that degree of force wasn't justified, or the entire fight wasn't justified, your new address is going to be Cell Block 25, D Wing. Cute comment aside, know that hitting this target carries with it some inherent risks. Be justified.

You are facing your opponent with your left leg forward when he throws a right front kick. You easily swat it aside and, before he can collect himself from the block, you step to your left with your left foot and whip your right shin into his floating ribs.

Practice 1 to 2 sets of 10 reps on both sides.

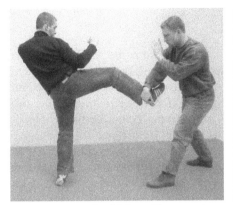 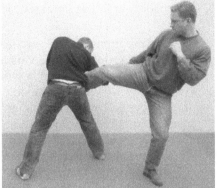

Parry the kick aside, step to your left and kick his floating ribs with your lower shin.

Keep these targets in mind as you practice with live partners and work the heavy bag. Remember that well-timed blows to the liver, solar plexus and the floating ribs are targets that have KOd many a fighter, even highly conditioned professionals. They are arguably better than hitting the head because there is less chance of breaking your hand, and the chance of debilitating an attacker is high, especially one with a soft gut.

When the attacker is wearing a heavy coat

There have been cases where a heavy winter coat has stopped a small caliber bullet. So unless you absolutely know that your punch or kick is more powerful, don't waste precious time and timing opportunities hitting into an attacker's coat.

While people typically wear big, bulky, well-padded coats in the winter, most wear jeans or slacks over their legs. Therefore, in foul weather, use your timing moments to attack the street thug's thighs, knees, shins and Achilles' tendons, or head hunt the eyes, ears, nose and throat.

High kicks in the street

"You *never* kick above the waist in a street fight."

"High kicks don't work because they are slow. They take more time to get to their target."

"High kicks aren't as powerful as low-line kicks."

How many times have you heard these statements when someone talks about sports fighting versus street defense? We have heard them countless times and disagree with all of them. Yes, you read that right: We disagree. Do we recommend using high kicks in a street fight? Yes and no. We recommend using the most appropriate technique for whatever specific situation you find yourself in. Though this seems like an evasive answer, it's just as we discussed in the beginning of this chapter: It's an "It depends" issue. Sometimes a fancy kick above the waist saves the day. Other times when you try to do it, your opponent crushes your testicles into a bloody mess with a well-placed front snap kick. Since things aren't always black and white, just keep in mind that sometimes it makes perfect sense to use a high kick. Here are a few examples:

- Earlier Demeere talked about using a high kick in a brawl to knock out his adversary.

- Demeere once knew a fighter who would learn a new technique and then go out and pick fights in bars to test it. He successfully used a variety of high kicks.

- One of Demeere's friends used to work as a bouncer. After the owner of the establishment had prohibited him from punching or head butting troublemakers, he switched to kicking them, using the lead-leg roundhouse to the head, as used often in point fighting. He would lean away from the rowdy customer, make a placating gesture to hide his weight transfer and then violently whip his kick into the man's head.

- Another bouncer acquaintance of Demeere's approached a group of rambunctious drinkers at a table. He tried negotiating, but it became clear they were interested only in tearing up the place. So the bouncer decided on a preemptive strike. He said, "Look, you guys gotta go," while leaning towards them with both hands on the table to stabilize his body. Then, so fast that no one could react, he whipped a roundhouse kick over the table, virtually in a full split at the completion of its arc, knocking unconscious a troublemaker who was about to jump him.

By no means do these stories prove high kicks are the best techniques for a street self-defense situation. But it does prove that *some* people can make them work in *some* situations. Each individual in these examples saw an opening and then used a technique they had trained on and had confidence in. Their actions defined the word "timing" as they took steps to overcome the inherent weakness of the high kick, in particular the lengthy travel time to get to the target, and then executed it perfectly through a window of opportunity.

The first bouncer leaned away from the threat and gestured with his hands as if to deny wanting to use force, a ruse designed to draw the man's attention away from his preparation to deliver the kick. The second bouncer placed his hands on a table and leaned in to close the distance with his target and camouflage that he was positioning his leg for the kick. By the time his kick launched over the table and was seen by the unruly customer (the lighting in the bar was poor, too), his leg was moving so fast that all the customer could do was get hit.

One other aspect, and one that is as important as perfect timing, is that all fighters had worked to develop knockout power with their kicks by training extensively on heavy bags and shields, and at full-contact sparring. This is in contrast to many flippy-dippy high kicks that earn points in non-contact tournaments, thrown by fighters who train mostly in the air, and only occasionally on the bags.

Here are a few questions to ask yourself before you launch a head-high kick in the street:

- How well can you execute a high kick? Are yours great or average? Don't lie to yourself now and then have self-doubt get in the way in a real situation. You need to be totally convinced that your high kicks are superior before using them in the real world.

- Are you extremely flexible? High kicks demand great flexibility. If you aren't flexible enough to perform high kicks when your muscles are cold, you should never use them in a real situation. There is no time to warm-up and stretch out when that thug is coming at you.

- Does your kick have enough "juice?" Throwing a quick and snappy point-fighting roundhouse kick might not do the damage needed to stop an attacker. Even if you are flexible, you must have power in your stretch to drive your foot, ankle or shin deep into the target, more power than is required for those controlled kicks used in point competition. This requires thousands of full-impact reps on the hand-helds and heavy bags to get the feel of your kicks and to understand your capability. If you can't deliver a powerful high kick, don't even think about using it to defend yourself.

- Are your kicks accurate? Most fighters can aim better with their punches and strikes than with their kicks, especially high kicks. You need to be able to consistently kick the neck, jaw, temple area, and ear as easily as you can punch them. A high kick that misses or glances off due to poor targeting can get you a laugh from the bad guy and then a sound trouncing.

To reiterate, you need to be able to kick high with blistering speed, hit with the impact of an elephant's stomp, possess impeccable timing, and have the confidence of Muhammad Ali in his prime. There is no room for error here. If you don't posses these qualities, then keep your kicks low.

We know it's controversial to say that some sport-fighting techniques are street applicable. To those who shake their head stubbornly and refuse to hear the argument, well, maybe they shouldn't dismiss a technique just because *they* can't do it. In this context, a person's inability to adapt a tournament technique to the street doesn't make it worthless for self-defense. We stand by our assertion that within the context we have discussed in this chapter and with all the qualifiers, many tournament techniques can be made to work in the real world. We have done it and we have seen others do it. However, doing so necessitates high-quality training, analytical study of what you are doing, confidence based on real skill, and a deep understanding of timing.

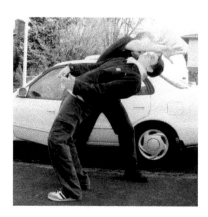

CHAPTER FIVE

TIMING A GRAB: CLOSE THE GAP

Not every confrontation is about kicking the adversary's teeth in.
Some are, but more aren't.

Let's talk about timing situations that don't call for you to hit the other person, but rather grab, push, or in some way put your hands on him. For example:

- Your brother-in-law has had too much too drink at the Christmas party and he is beginning to get a little ugly with it. You want to take him out on the porch for air.

- A patron is causing a disturbance at a bar or restaurant. You want to get him out the door before he gets physical.

- An angry motorist is standing next to your car and not letting you in.

- You are a football referee and an angry parent has confronted you in the parking lot.

In all of these situations, you must cross that very dangerous space between you and the subject without getting force-fed a knuckle sandwich. It's not always easy to do, but it's easier when you time it right.

Law enforcement needs this, too

As a police officer or security officer, you know how to apply a couple of wristlocks and an elbow press, and you can keep a squirrelly suspect under control while you slap on the handcuffs. But few academies teach the importance of how to cross the space between you and a prison-hard ex-convict who wants some payback for all that time he sat in stir. This is a glaring omission. It doesn't matter how many neat-o techniques you know, because if you can't cross those two or three steps to the suspect without getting punched, you might not get a chance to use them. Instead, you become a member of the Assaulted Officers Club, an organization that boasts (well, maybe not "boasts") a membership of hundreds of thousands of police and security officers every year.

To reduce the chance of membership, it's imperative that you follow the advice throughout this book, particularly in this chapter. Now, if you are no longer the young cowboy you were as a rookie 15 years ago, and you aren't in the best physical condition, you will find that these techniques and gimmicks work great (to get in the best physical condition, check out our book *The Fighter's Body: An Owner's Manual*. Sorry, couldn't resist). Know that with just a little physical practice at crossing the gap, you dramatically reduce the chance of getting punched in the nose. The better you are at anything that helps you go home at the end of your shift builds your confidence and comforts to your partner and family.

Let's examine a car break-in scenario, something that happens thousands of times every day. While the following is presented for analysis by people who aren't police officers, those readers who are should study them from the standpoint of law enforcement needs.

The setting

You are on a downtown sidewalk standing about six feet away from a guy who just scooted out of your car as you walked up. He is clearly drunk and clearly holding your stereo. You call to a passerby to phone 9-1-1 and then think quickly about how you are going to prevent the thief from leaving, since either by his words or actions, it's clear that he isn't going to wait around for the gendarmes. Now, you don't have a legal right to smash him in the face, but you can hold him for the police. To do so, you have to safely cross the space between you. You can simply cross that gap into his striking range and hope that you react in time to whatever action he takes or, better yet, you can time your move to when he is vulnerable physically, mentally or both.

Let's examine briefly eight moments in time, or windows of opportunity, when the thief is most vulnerable to you crossing the gap. In all of these, you must move with speed because perfect timing means taking advantage of a moment, a moment that may last no longer than half a second.

Those old tricks of yours

If you have other gap-crossing timing tricks that have worked for you in the past, don't throw them away. We do encourage you to analyze them and see how they fit in with other concepts discussed in this chapter and throughout the book. Yours might have worked out of luck or out of absolute genius on your part. Those that involve mostly luck, dissect to see if they can be fixed so they are based on sound concepts and principles. If they can't be fixed, it's probably best to set them on the back burner and call on them only when all else fails. With those that are sound, grab a training partner and use the practice methods at the end of this chapter to improve them even more.

Though your objective is to cross the gap between you and the thief, a space that sometimes seems like a yawning canyon, and apply a restraint hold, there is always the chance you might have to defend against a sudden and explosive punch. These eight gap-closing methods reduce that possibility. *Reduces*, not eliminates.

1. Move when he is distracted

This is arguably one of the easiest times to move against a hostile suspect. The distraction may be a natural one: a honking horn from a passing car, a noisy airplane, the roar of an accelerating city bus, a passerby asking what you are doing, or a ray of sun suddenly piercing through a cloud.

You can also create a distraction, most often by something you say to him.

"Oh good, here comes the police car."

"Here comes my buddy, the weight lifting champion. You're not going to like him."

"Is that your car over there?" Even if they don't have a car, they look.

"Do you know that pretty lady (handsome guy)?"

This form of distraction works best when you first pretend to "see" the thing or person, and then make your statement or ask the question. For example, look over his shoulder for a split second, widen your eyes a little, and then say your line.

Even if he turns only part way before it dawns on him that you're just being a trickster, that is usually sufficient distraction to allow you to charge across the gap. For him to react to you, he has to process through his OODA loop: He has to turn back in your direction; it has to register in his mind that it's not a good thing that you are charging toward him; he has to think how to respond; and then he has to put that response into action. Yes, he can do all this quickly, but it provides you with just enough time to cross that space.

2. When he changes stances

We discussed this technique earlier, but let's revisit it using our car prowler scenario.

As you talk to the guy, you notice that he is nervous or high on something, as he continually changes his stance from his left foot forward to his right, shifting his weight each time. He turns part way around and then turns back to face you. It's almost as if he is displaying awkward stances as an invitation for you to charge him. So you do. .

Just as he begins to switch from one position to the next – say, by stepping back with his lead leg – explode forward with all the speed you can muster. You didn't telegraph your charge, did you? Extend your arms in front of you to protect yourself and grab his closest arm, shoulder, wrist or whatever you can get. If he is turned part way around, push him the rest of the way so that his back is to you and then take him to the ground, or push him up against the side of the car.

If you have a sharp eye and notice that his weight is mostly on one leg, say his right one, push him to the right. His unbalanced stance, even when mildly unbalanced, makes it much easier to take him to the ground.

Practice 1 to 2 sets of 10 reps on both sides.

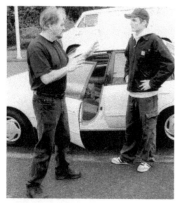
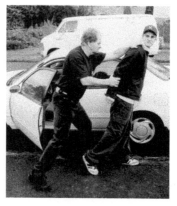

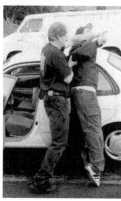

As you talk to the thief, he turns part way around providing you with an opportunity to lunge at him, then jam him against the car with an arm lock and head press.

3. Catch him with his feet parallel

The thief's stance is also weak when he stands with his feet shoulder width apart, toes pointed at you. This is an awkward position to fight from because he needs to shift his weight to one leg before he can act offensively or defensively. He is strongest when his body is turned at an angle to you and his feet are staggered, the stance assumed by most boxers and karate people, a solid position from which he can fire off a quick attack.

So, if he assumes the feet parallel stance, even for a second, it's incumbent upon you to grab at that moment by lunging forward and knocking him off his perch. He might step back reflexively with one foot in response to you, but it's not going to make much difference if your gap closing technique is fast. Now, should he realize his foot position error about the same time you notice, it will take him a half second to modify it. As already discussed, moving in on him when he changes stances is also a good timing moment. *Practice 1 to 2 sets of 10 reps on both sides.*

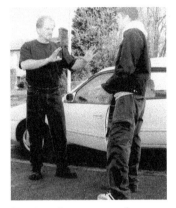 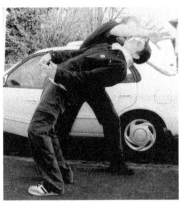

During the course of your confrontation, the thief brings both his feet parallel with each other. That is the perfect moment to charge him with a clothesline forearm across his neck or face.

4. When he drops his hands

Your objective with this timing method is to catch the suspect with his arms in a weak position. When he lowers them to his sides, fists his hands on his hips or tries to look bored with you by plunging them into his pockets, those are weak positions, weak moments that should be exploited. Be cognizant of his hands as you move in, as most likely they will react to your sudden lunge. But if you time it right and move with good speed, his reaction will be too late. *Practice 1 to 2 sets of 10 reps on both sides.*

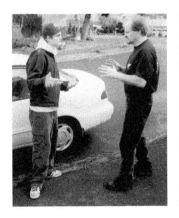 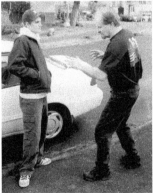

He has his hands in front of him as he speaks. The moment he plunges them into his pockets, move in.

5. When moving back

Here are a couple of facts about moving backward that you can use to your advantage. You can move forward faster than the thief can move backward; few people can scramble backward more than two or three steps without tripping and falling down. Christensen once trained with one of Bruce Lee's students, a man who was extraordinarily fast and could cross the gap like a bullet. He picked several black belts out of the group and charged each one, one at a time. He told them not to counter but rather scramble back as fast as they could. Each one tried and each one went sprawling on the floor. Now, if this happened to highly-trained fighters, imagine what would happen to your drunk car prowler.

Let's say in the course of your contact with the person that you notice whenever you gesture toward him or move ever so slightly in his direction, he spooks backward a step or two. This is good.

Try maneuvering him so that there is a curb, fire hydrant, park bench or parked car directly to his rear (no, you can't use a passing train). When the moment is right, lunge toward him. If he responds as he has before, he will scramble backwards right into, or over, whatever is in his path. While he struggles to recover, a moment that may last only a couple of seconds, that is your opportunity to move in and gain control of him.

 Not all is lost if the two of you are standing in an open field or on an empty parking lot where there are no obstacles to make him stumble. It's imperative, however, that you charge him hard and fast so that he reacts in a startle mode. Most people will trip after about three steps, especially if they are not athletic or are under the influence of something.

Don't stop after the initial two or three strides because an astute thief will take one additional step back, turn and run off. To minimize this from happening, charge him fast and don't stop until you catch him.

One other caution is to be careful not to trip over the suspect. If you are almost on him and he stumbles and falls onto his back, you're susceptible to getting entangled in his legs and falling onto him. Watch him carefully. When he starts to go down, angle off to the right or left so that you avoid his plight.

Practice 1 to 2 sets of 10 reps.

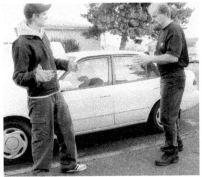 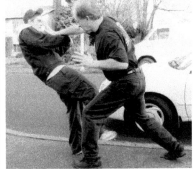

You notice the thief keeps stepping back nervously. Seize the moment to force him back until he stumbles and falls.

6. When he retracts his attack

Okay, let's kick up the intensity a little. Your contact with the guy deteriorates suddenly – it occurs to his small brain that he is going to miss out on breaking into lots more cars if he is in jail— and he throws a punch at you. It misses or just grazes your iron jaw. Once he launches his punch and it hits or misses, his arm starts retracting, and unless he is a highly trained martial artist it's no longer of immediate concern to you. That is when you make your move. It's a window of opportunity that lasts only a second so don't hesitate. *Practice 1 to 2 sets of 10 reps on both sides.*

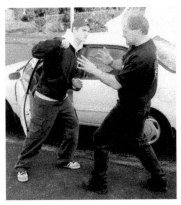 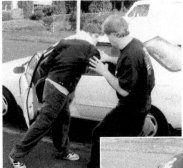

The car thief swings at you and you brush it by. Take advantage of his unbalance to grab the back of his neck and arm to drive him to the sidewalk.

War story   A doped-up street prostitute once took a wild swing at Christensen. He leaned back just enough to let the arc pass by his nose without connecting, and then he pushed her upper arm to force her body to continue turning until her back was to him. Then he dumped her on the sidewalk.

7. When he is talking

While this method sometimes works when you are two or three paces away from a slow-to-respond person, it's most effective when you are just a tad outside of his arm's reach. This is because typically a person's reaction time with this one is faster than with the others.

Let's say you are dealing with someone on the verge of exploding. Every muscle in his body has gone rigid, his hands are fisted along his sides, his neck cords are bulging, and his eyes are boring into you. For your technique to work, you must employ two principles: action/reaction, a moment where reaction is slower than action, and distraction, a moment where a person can think of only one thing at a time.

Note: We are talking about an entirely different level of force here, one in which you could legally punch or kick, that is, should you decide to move against a person in such a state of mind. Legal-wise and safety-wise, it might be best to let him go and give the police a good physical description and the direction he fled. But for the sake of discussing this concept, let's continue.

Your objective is to get the person to talk so that he has to first think about what he wants to say and then articulate it. That process, though done quickly, occupies his mind. For him to react to you reaching toward his arm, to you swatting aside his weapon, or to you pushing him backwards, he has to *see* your action, *stop talking* to *clear* his mind so he can *define* what your action means, *decide* how to react, and then *do* so in some fashion. In other words, he has to begin a new OODA loop (see Chapter One). If he is under the influence, it might take him a tad longer to get through the loop, maybe a whole extra second, which is even better for you.

It also works when it's you doing the talking because his mind has to work to understand what he is hearing you say. To react to your action, he has to switch mental gears. It's arguably more effective when the personis talking, but you are encouraged to try both in your training since you might have to face a someone who won't say a word, thus forcing you to do all the talking.

8. When you are with a buddy

In a perfect world, you and your buddy recognize the timing moment at the same time and launch yourselves simultaneously at the thief like a fine-tuned machine. However, since it's an imperfect world, more than likely only one of you will recognize the opportunity and move, or both of you will see it, but one will move before the other.

War story: Christensen and his police partner were talking to an agitated and distraught teenage boy at a domestic violence call. In the blink of an eye, the kid lunged for a rifle that had been placed out of sight behind a door. Christensen moved first and grabbed the kid's throat from the front in a claw choke. A hair of an instant later his partner moved behind the kid and wrapped his beefy arm around the boy's neck in a more conventional carotid artery hold. Since Christensen's hand was already on the kid's neck, his hand got trapped under his partner's arm. It took a couple of embarrassing seconds to free his hand, but at least no one got shot.

One of you moving first can be a big problem if the other doesn't follow. If your buddy suddenly lunges across the space toward the guy, you should immediately follow, understanding that he must have seen something even if you didn't. This works smoothly when the two of you have an understanding of timing opportunities, and agree that should you get into a situation together, and one moves suddenly, the other should follow.

Here is a simple way you can split the thief's attention when he is standing at 12 o'clock, you are standing at 8 o'clock and your buddy is at 4. From this classic position, you can apply any of the above timing opportunities, or try this one.

When the person looks at the one speaking, the other lunges across the gap. When the bad guy reacts to him, then the other one charges forward.

OODA loop revisited Know that when you decide to cross the gap to grab someone, your speed is determined by how fast you go through the OODA loop.

- **Observe:** You observe the thief's actions

- **Orient:** You note his position in relation to you and the rest of the setting.

- **Decide:** You select the right technique for the moment.

- **Act on the Decision:** You put into action your selected technique -- lunge and grab his arm; lunge and push him; lunge and tackle him -- as fast as you are able.

Training ideas

The instructor groups the students into pairs and then has them decide amongst themselves who will be the bad guy and who will be the angry victim of a car break-in. Begin with the first timing drill discussed in this article: "When he is distracted."

The victim says something to distract the bad guy, and the bad guy reacts by looking away, or turning partially or all the way around. The good guy then seizes the moment and lunges forward to apply a control hold.

After both students have practiced being the good guy, the instructor progresses to the next technique discussed in this article, "When he drops his hands." Again, each student gets to play the good guy, before progressing to the next timing method. If the instructor or students have other effective timing methods not discussed here, those should be included in the workout, too.

Besides moving at the right time and with all-out speed, the instructor should watch the good guys to ensure they aren't telegraphing their intentions. He should watch for sharp breath inhalations, tugging at a pant leg, shrugging the shoulders, twitching the mouth, or shouting, "Here I come!" (Just kidding about the last one.)

In all of these, the bad guy should let the good guy win since the drill is to develop the various phases that make up timing speed; it's not about fighting a resisting person. Once the instructor feels the students have established good timing, he can then make the exercise more complex, including having the bad guys resist when the good guys lunge in.

Practice 1 to 2 sets of 10 reps on both sides of all the drills.

Not every confrontation is about kicking the adversary's teeth in. Some are, but more aren't. If you can close the gap and apply a control hold to restrain a person until help arrives or the authorities show up, you have handled the situation wisely, responsibly, and without risk of lawsuit.

Doing your civic duty

You might suddenly find yourself in the middle of a situation where you can assist law enforcement. If you choose to act as a good citizen and help, it's nice to know how. Christensen says that there were many times as a police officer when he was alone and struggling with a resistor when someone stepped out of the crowd and helped take the person to the ground. In fact, Christensen has a picture taken from the newspaper of him in uniform applying an armbar technique to a violent protestor's left arm and a man in civilian clothes applying the same technique to the protestor's other arm. Christensen says that he was having trouble getting the big man down when the Good Samaritan stepped out of the crowd and applied a hold to help drop the protestor onto his belly. The man's technique was flawless and he appeared to have been trained. As soon as Christensen applied the handcuffs, his helper blended back into the crowd, never to be seen again.

Since you never know, be prepared.

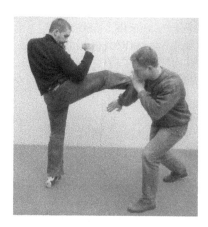

CHAPTER SIX

WISDOM OF THE AGES

Success comes from constant training, constant examination of yourself, and constant examination of your material. This is where the classics can help

As a martial arts student, police officer, or professional military officer, chances are you have studied such great reads as *The Art of War*, by Sun Tzu, *A Book of Five Rings* by Miyamoto Musashi, and the so-called Tai Chi Chuan Classics. If you have not read any of them, know that they are a necessity in every thinking fighter's library. These Classics aren't the books you pick up when you want an entertaining, easy-to-read novel. Think of them as scholarly bibles of the fighting arts, books meant to be studied over and over, as you cross-reference knowledge from several areas of your training and then place that knowledge into a bigger context as presented in these books. You just might find, as many other fighters have, that by examining ways to combine your knowledge with information in these Classics, many aspects of your fighting skill will change for the better: timing, footwork, the way in which specific techniques are executed, and why you use them in specific instances. The Classics might improve little details in your fight game and other times they might reveal a whole new range of possibilities. Sometimes it's the small details that are crucial to your victory in a life and death situation; other times it's the big epiphanies. Both can be found in the classics.

"To study" comes from the Latin verb *studere*, which means "to be eager," or "to apply oneself." To learn from the Classics requires that you have a drive to learn combined with willingness to continuously re-examine your knowledge throughout the years. This means that as you go through your cycles of training – growth spurts, plateaus, injuries, boredom, enthusiasm, leaning new material, epiphanies – you will reread these books with new understanding, new depth, and newfound wisdom that affects positively the quality of your training and quality of your skills.

Though we feel the Classics have invaluable wisdom for both sports martial arts and self-defense, particularly in the area of timing, understand that you aren't going to find in them secret keys that unlock the total potential of all your techniques, making them "100 percent guaranteed or your money back!" Sadly, there are no such shortcuts to martial arts success. Success comes from constant training, constant examination of yourself, and constant examination of your material. This is where the Classics can help.

The challenge

The challenge is to understand what you read and then apply the information. Admittedly, that is no small feat. As with all translations, it's incredibly difficult not to lose information when transposing text from one language to another: some words can't be translated because they don't exist in the other language; words or sentences carry connotations and implications too subtle to translate without adding a volume of footnotes; the translator may lack the experience as a warrior or martial artist to bring across what the author means; the author might mention a concept that doesn't exist in the other culture's language or, if it does, it means something different.

To complicate things further, the Classics were written hundreds of years ago in the Orient. Not only is there a world of difference between English/Anglo-Saxon cultures and Japanese and Chinese cultures, but there is a huge time gap between most current translations and the era in which these classics were written. This makes much of it difficult to read, especially since the original texts used a type of archaic writing style modern readers are unaccustomed to.

The good news

Despite these issues, the Classics are still invaluable for today's warriors. Every day, the strategies, concepts and critical analysis in them prove viable on battlefields around the world, in one-on-one fighting competition, in street self-defense, and even in the business world where individuals and companies battle each other in charged competition. Why, after hundreds of years, is the material not only still relevant, but highly relevant? Simple. At the time they were written, just as now, all men and women had two arms and two legs attached to a torso with a head on top. Therefore, what was true principle-wise, concept-wise, and strategy-wise in those violent times still holds valuable lessons for our era's violence, though you might have to make adjustments and adaptations here and there. They force you to not only study their meanings on an intellectual level, but to physically practice their concepts, as well. It's in this training, the physical and the skull sweat, where you enhance your skills and knowledge. The information is there. All you need to do to make it yours is work hard.

The Tai Chi Chuan Classics

The Tai Chi Classics are an ensemble of five essays, usually attributed to Chang San-feng, recognized by many schools as the founder of tai chi, though there are some who debate this. Parts of the Classics cover philosophy and specific information for tai chi chuan practitioners, and there is also great advice regarding timing applicable for any martial art. Consider the following excerpts, as translated by tai chi chuan expert Dan Docherty:

> *From the feet to the legs through the waist, all must be completely uniform and, simultaneous, whether stepping forward or moving back. This will result in good timing and correct movements.*

> *If in certain places good timing and correct body movement are not achieved, body movements become arbitrary and disordered. This sickness must be sought in the waist and in the legs.*

What this means

In tai chi chuan and many other martial arts, you want to move your body as a connected whole, as opposed to moving its parts separately. By timing your movements so that every part of your body starts and stops at the same time, you are able to put your entire bodyweight into your technique, thus increasing its power many times over. Though there are other ways of generating power, this method doesn't rely on raw muscle strength, good news for smaller fighters or those lacking physical strength.

But don't you always move the weapon first?

While it might appear that there is a conflict in the way tai chi moves as opposed to the often-taught concept of moving the weapon first, there isn't. The goal in tai chi is to coordinate the body with the attack to get more mass behind it. Though the attacking limb and the body start moving at the same time, that doesn't mean they move at the same speed. The arm may appear to be moving earlier than the body, but the body has already started moving a little. The main difficulty is to ensure they both stop moving at the same time. That way, your full energy is behind the punch or kick, so that the technique doesn't end up being a feeble pushing action. It takes lots of practice, but once learned, it generates great power in every offensive action.

There is a natural tendency for novice fighters to try and use sheer muscle to increase the power of a technique, usually by contracting their arm and upper body muscles as hard as they can. The tai chi classics clearly warn to avoid this by using coordinated movement, specifically, drawing power from your legs and transferring it via the waist to the limbs. Try this:

Block and punch   Your partner throws a reverse punch at your face, which you avoid by leaning away, stepping to your left, and parrying with the back of your right arm. Then step toward him, pushing off your support leg as you continue to push his attacking arm aside, and put your entire body weight behind a pile-driving left reverse punch into his ribs. The key is this: Once you start moving, transfer the energy from your legs to your punching arm by means of a tight twist of your waist. With practice, you can land a blow that coordinates both the stepping and the waist turning with the punch so they all come together at one moment, a moment that breaks your opponent's ribs.

Practice 1 or 2 sets of 10 reps on both sides.

The Tai Chi Classics say:

> *"If the opponent's actions are swift then my response is swift. If his actions are slow then I slowly follow them."*

What this means

This quote clearly recommends that your timing match your attacker's moves, specifically his speed. Concentrating on his actions and adapting to them gives you more options to use against him than you would have if you were focused only on what you want to do to him. Also, it reduces the chance of being blindsided or making a poor judgment call. Ignore this simple advice from the classics and you risk being faced with two major timing problems: timing your technique too soon, so that he sees it and easily counters you, or timing it too late, which makes it ineffective and allows him the opportunity to lands his attack. Try this:

Fluctuating speed drill After you and your training partner assume your fighting stances, he launches five repetitions of a medium speed reverse punch. You in return respond five times with a parry and body evasion combination. Your partner then increases the speed in small increments, after every fifth rep, until the two of you are going full speed. Once you are comfortable at high speeds, your partner changes his attacking mode to one of random speed: sometimes he throws a scorching-fast punch, then a slow one, and then one at medium speed. While this isn't difficult, you have to pay attention so you don't execute your defense too soon and leave yourself wide open, or respond too late should his suddenly fast punch catch you off guard.

Practice 1 set of 15 reps: 5 slow, 5 medium, and 5 fast.

Practice 1 set of 10 reps at random speed.

The Tai Chi Classics say:

"Many err by forsaking what is near to pursue what is far"

What this means

We mention this elsewhere in this book and have picked this quote to underscore the point. Many fighters, especially those with little experience, not only pick the wrong techniques given the timing moment, but they try for targets that aren't accessible right then, or try to use techniques that are too complicated, take too long to pull off, or are strategically not a good idea. Christensen likes to say that there are no absolutely wrong choices, but there are many that are much better. Consider these examples:

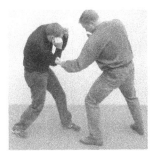

- Say your attacker has assumed a tight boxing-type guard with his ribs and midsection protected by his forearms and elbows. If you try to land a direct hit there, you are likely to bang uselessly on his arms and leave yourself wide open for a devastating counter. (The exception here is when you are punching at his arms deliberately to weaken and injure them. For our purposes in this example, we are referring to fighters who punch them out of frustration and poor target selection.)

- You punch at his face when his head is too far away even to kick, forcing you to lean into your strike and over commit your balance.

- You are in a clinch and your opponent has your arms restrained. You struggle to punch him, though he is ripe for a knee strike.

These happen because you aren't alert to what your opponent is doing, and you aren't thinking clearly about where he is open or what technique is best for the timing moment. This quote advises to keep things simple and direct, never go for the fancy or spectacular. Punching at a too-far-away target, or trying to use a limb that is being restrained isn't taking advantage of a timing moment; it's wasting time and doing so dangerously.

Statue: One of the best drills we know to remedy this problem is the drill "Statue," described in Chapter Two. It specifically forces you to look for openings from wherever you may find yourself, rather than flailing madly in hopes of hitting something.

CHAPTER 6 ───────────────────────────

The Art of War

This classic, written well over 2000 years ago and attributed to a general named Sun Tzu, was originally intended as a manual for military leaders in ancient China. It has been studied throughout the years for military purposes and, in recent years, its strategies and tactics have been used by businesses ranging from one-person stores to multinational corporations, all with great results. Let's consider three quotes from The Art of War that relate to timing.

> *"Thus the highest form of generalship is to balk the enemy's plans; the next best is to prevent the junction of the enemy's forces; the next in order is to attack the enemy's army in the field; and the worst policy of all is to besiege walled cities.*

What this means

This is a powerful quote, whether as an overall strategy for war, with armies, tanks and falling bombs, or when defending yourself all by your lonesome against a vicious street fighter. There is no argument that the best way to win a confrontation is to not engage in it at all. As we have discussed earlier, it's best to use alertness and awareness to identify and avoid potential trouble, verbal judo to talk your way out of a situation, or to seek an avenue of escape and run like the wind.

When prevention fails, it's time to rumble. Because you know there is no other way out of the situation, you are psychologically prepared for battle. You have analyzed the situation to form a plan using your well-honed skills, and the many concepts and tricks described throughout this book.

You must never waste energy fighting your opponent's strong points. If he has a solid defense and you know he is a powerful counter puncher, don't storm into him as if you were a battering ram trying to crash through the gates of a fortress. It's better to look for weak spots where your attacks would be more effective: knees, shins, even his forearms. An underlying skill of every successful military strategist or street fighter is knowing how to be selective with the available resources. Don't waste them on actions that are futile, as you risk running out of energy or leaving yourself wide open to his nasty counter punch.

Instead of discussing a single move, that wouldn't do the text justice, let's apply the lesson to a modern-day scenario. Let's break the quote into its three sentences.

> "Thus the highest form of generalship is to balk the enemy's plans"

You notice a few feet ahead of you on the sidewalk, a tough-looking, muscular street person eyeing you as you approach. You cross the street to avoid contact and thus "balk the enemy's plans."

> "The next best is to prevent the junction of the enemy's forces"

The thug quickly crosses, blocks your avenue of escape and starts cussing and screaming. You try verbal judo, being careful to stay out of his reach, while keeping an eye out for a potential second thug ambushing from behind.

> "The next in order is to attack the enemy's army in the field and the worst policy of all is to besiege walled cities"

He screams a final obscenity and launches a jab-cross combination. Since you were mentally prepared for the attack, you quickly sidestep and dodge the punches. While staying out of punching range (which you know from his attack is his strong point), you land a vicious sidekick to his knee, knocking him down so that you can run to safety.

Here is another quote from Sun Tzu.

> "What enables an army to withstand the enemy's attack and not be defeated are uncommon and common maneuvers."

What this means

A fighter needs to be flexible and adaptable as the situation evolves. If you go into a fight assuming it's going to be an easy win because your killer kung fu kick is impossible to block, you are likely to get hurt. The only thing you should assume is that it's seldom a good idea to make assumptions. Stay alert for the inevitability of change. This quote makes a case for not only training hard on your commonly known and often used techniques -- your basic kicks and punches -- but also to work hard on uncommon ones for purposes of surprise.

Since there is a counter for every technique, it's possible your opponent can counter your common attack but will have trouble countering what is uncommon, those techniques that make him wonder, "What was that?" Now, don't read into this that you have to invent weird and impractical techniques to make this concept work, because you don't.

Uncommon additions Try spitting at your opponent before you launch a round kick into his groin (clearly we are talking about the street here, not competition); scream like a female actress in a horror movie just before you backfist him; wave "hi" with your fingers to make him go "Huh?" just before you kick him in the groin. By combining both common and uncommon techniques, you apply flexibility, adaptability and creativity to help prevail in a wide variety of violent situations.

Practice 1 or 2 sets of 10 reps on both sides. Suggestion: Simulate the spitting.

Sun Tzu says:

> "The rush of torrential waters tossing boulders illustrates force. The strike of a bird of prey breaking the body of its target illustrates timing. Therefore, the force of those skilled in warfare is overwhelming, and their timing precise. Their force is like a drawn crossbow and their timing is like the release of the trigger."

What this means

Let's define "torrential waters" as a large mass of water rolling over everything with such forward momentum that it sweeps away anything not strong enough to resist. While water in great volume has an ever-changing form, depending on what it must adapt to or what it encounters in its path, its mass sustains its tremendous energy. When fighting, you want to be like that torrential mass of water. You want unstoppable power to overwhelm your opponent as you push forward with aggression, all the while adapting to the situation as needed.

A "bird of prey" takes to the skies and then goes into a nosedive, gathering incredible speed to strike its unsuspecting victim on the ground. It has to time its flight exactly right or it will miss the target and crash into the dirt. This analogy shows how nature combines overwhelming force (the bird going 100mph) and perfect timing (it must adjust its flight path to catch the prey) to defeat a specific target. You want to do exactly the same thing when you fight.

The next sentence of the quote joins unstoppable force and precise timing. Your powerful techniques are useless if you can't time them to hit a target. On the flip side, perfect timing with weak blows are equally useless.

The last sentence offers advice on a technical and psychological level. It means that a crossbow is ready to destroy when the string is drawn back, and to hit the target, one must aim with precision and then release the trigger at the correct time. Likewise, for you to overwhelm your attacker, you must execute techniques that have as much power as possible, and deliver them at the absolute best moment. To develop this ability, you must develop good form, shave off excess movement, and practice the many timing drills and concepts in this book. To achieve a mind-set capable of unleashing tremendous force as fast as the blink of an eye at the right moment, you must train hard. Very hard. There is no way around this.

Lift and throw Face your opponent just outside of kicking range and wait for his attack. As he launches a hard front kick, step to the side and scoop it up in the crook of your arm. Without pausing, lift his leg higher and higher as you drive forward, adding your entire body to the momentum, like that giant torrential wave, and keep going until your charge and his elevated leg causes him to lose balance and fall onto his head, hard.

Practice 1 or 2 sets of 10 reps on both sides.

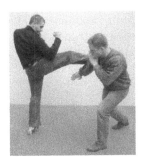 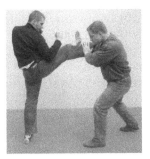 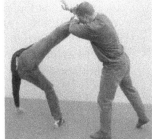

Block and scoop your opponent's kick, then lift his leg toss him onto his head.

A Book of Five Rings

Miyamoto Musashi, a Japanese warrior born in the 16th century, wrote *A Book of Five Rings*, a treatise on strategy, after studying and living it his entire life. He killed his first opponent in a duel at age 13 and went on to use his sword to strike down over 60 others. He is considered by many to be most famous samurai in history. Let's look at three passages from A Book of Five Rings that relate to timing.

> *"Whether you move fast or slow, with large or small steps, your feet must always move as in normal walking."*

> *"Yin-Yang foot means not moving only one foot."*

What this means

Musashi suggests using natural footwork when fighting, as opposed to using overly complicated footwork patterns or jumping around as seen so often in modern karate tournaments.

When you walk, your left foot follows your right, and so on until you get to your destination. Okay, you already knew that, but also know that you should move the same way in a fight. When moving to the left, your left leg moves first, followed by your right. Seldom, if ever, should you cross your legs, do a fancy twirl, or summersault. And, contrary to modern kata competition, there are few times when fighting to save your face would you ever do a cartwheel or leap into the air and land in a split. Simple, natural footwork is economical and, therefore, a quick and smooth way to move both offensively and defensively.

Musashi says "…not moving only one foot," meaning, one leg follows the other. This was crucial in his days when defending against long blades that could slice through stone. If a samurai were to lean away from a downward cut by stepping sideways with just one leg, he would save his upper body from being split in half. But unless he executed a simultaneous deflection or attack with his sword, his attacker's weapon would continue its downward motion and slice neatly through the leg he didn't move.

While the chance of having to defend yourself against a sword today is slim (incredibly, it does happen from time to time), you are more likely to have to defend against a baseball bat or tire iron. Moving only one leg and leaving your other in the line of fire of your assailant's strike isn't a wise battle plan.

A final lesson in Musashi's writing is that you should train to fight from a natural position, one you use when just standing around. Some attacks happen so suddenly that you won't have time to drop into a wide Bruce Lee-like stance or the classic quarter turn, hands up fighting posture. It's just smart training to practice from a variety of natural positions: feet parallel with your body facing the threat; left lead; right lead; feet shoulder width apart; wider; when stepping; seated, and so on. The idea is to train in these positions so that in time all postures can be considered a fighting stance.

Here is how a nice timing moment, an opportunity to counter your opponent, can fail when you move only one leg.

Step and counter: Your opponent throws a right reverse punch. You step sideways with your left leg with the thought of driving a fast palm-heel strike into his ear, since his extended arm has left it open. When his punch misses you, he loses his balance and falls forward, and instinctively tries to recover from the forward momentum by taking a few quick steps. But because you didn't move your right leg when your left foot stepped, he slams into it, knocking you to the floor, too. A wonderful timing moment disrupted, and now you are in a ground-fighting situation. The outcome would have been much better had you followed Musashi's advice and moved both legs.

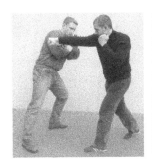
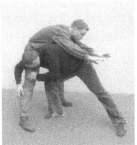
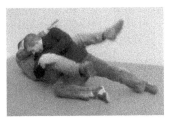

The wrong way is to step to your left and leave your right leg extended (above) because your opponent could lose his balance and fall into your leg, taking you with him. The right way is to side step with both feet and counter attack (right).

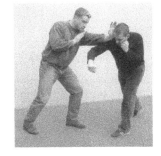

"When the enemy attacks, remain undisturbed but feign weakness. As the enemy reaches you, suddenly move away, indicating that you intend to jump aside, then dash in attacking strongly as soon as you see the enemy relax."

What this means

This strategy is based on two main concepts: deception and perfect timing. First, you bait your opponent into attacking and then pretend to be too hurt or too scared to do something about it. Though he might remain alert, it's human nature for him to mentally relax a tad when he perceives your display of what appears to be cowardice or injury. Seeing you in this condition gives him a sense of superiority, which often leads the less experienced fighter into complacency.

The next part is to reinforce that sense of overconfidence. As he moves in to attack you, step away as if too frightened to mount an offensive. Your objective here is to get him to provide you with a small window of opportunity when he relaxes his attentiveness even more as he begins to savor his victory. Now, don't laugh out loud in front of him quite yet. Instead, take advantage of this fleeting moment, this timing moment brought to you by Musashi, and strike him down with a furious attack to wherever he is open. This requires a cool head, some acting skills, and precise timing on your part. Here is how you can make this a result-producing training drill.

Feign and fight: As your training partner verbally abuses you and sets up his attack, lean away, put up your hands in the I-don't-want-to-fight stance, widen your eyes in fear, and plead for him not to hurt you. Make it believable. As soon as he steps into range with his false confidence, step back to reinforce your vulnerability in his mind. He will probably try to close the distance again, so you again step back. Then you attack.

When you take that second step, don't just plant your foot backwards but stomp it down to explode forwards into your unsuspecting opponent with a hard palm-heel to his face. Think of the footwork as what happens when you bounce a rubber ball against a wall: In a fraction of a second, the ball changes from going one direction to accelerating in another. Same with your foot. One instant you are stepping away from him, and the next you are storming forward to knock him down. If you can step at an angle when you move back, you force him to change directions as he advances, which provides you with a hair of a second more time to slam into him, making it even more difficult for him to defend.

It's critical to pay close attention to his response as you set him up so you can surprise him just when he thinks he has you beat. Remember what Musashi said: "As soon as you see the enemy relax," strike him down.

Practice 1 or 2 sets of 10 reps on both sides.

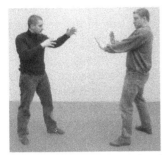 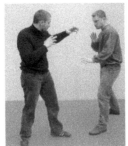 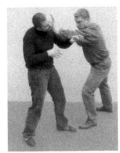

Feign fear and step back. Step another step back at an angle and then bounce forward to strike.

"In single combat, also you must put yourself in the enemy's position. If you think, 'Here is a master of the Way, who knows the principles of strategy', then you will surely lose."

What this means

When two people face each other in preparation to do combat, both experience an adrenaline rush and a boiling pot of stress. One of the most common reactions of the inexperienced fighter is to see the opponent as more than he is -- taller, stronger and meaner -- which only increases his fear and makes it harder to mount a defense. Should this happen to you, know that the longer it goes on, the worse it gets, because it creates a vicious circle. You feel intimidated and start doubting yourself, which causes more fear and results in more physical indicators of stress: weak knees, lightheadedness and tunnel vision. This in turn makes you doubt even more and the circle begins again, but with greater intensity. By the time your opponent hits you, you have already defeated yourself by all that is going on in your head.

Part of this problem is caused by the natural psychological and physiological reactions we have when faced with violence (for greater detail, check out *Deadly Force Encounters* by Loren W. Christensen and Dr. Alexis Artwohl). Knowing this won't help unless you take preventative measures in your training *before* you are faced with that proverbial ugly, giant, iron pumping, ex-con. You need to include stress in your training to become familiar with the adrenaline surge and that herd of butterflies in your stomach, reactions that can send the untrained down a mental spiral of fear and insecurity. Stress training is done mainly when practicing scenarios, as discussed in Chapter One, where training partners act out anxiety-producing situations. Going through these over and over again teaches you to deal with stress so that it doesn't paralyze you. This won't make fighting any less dangerous but since you are more prepared mentally, it will increase your chance of getting out in one piece.

One other element of this quote is to consider what the confrontation feels like to your opponent. He might look intimidating but that doesn't mean he is confident. Even big, muscular men can feel insecure, especially if they have never fought before. It might even be argued that they have more to lose ego-wise because of how they look and because of an expectation they will win. What Musashi says is to put yourself in the other man's shoes and realize that he too is experiencing an adrenaline dump into his system, since he doesn't know who you are or your capabilities.

A final point is that you need to analyze and try to predict how your opponent will act. This doesn't mean you have to be psychic (though that would be helpful). Neither can you make an assumption about him and then be oblivious to all the other possibilities he has (refer to "Mushin" in Chapter One). Instead, try to size him up and determine his strong points so you can put together a battle plan. Does he move like an experienced fighter or is he more "wooden?" Is he light and quick on his feet (perhaps favoring kicks) or more firmly planted on the ground (boxer/grappler)?

Scenario training   Devise several stress-producing scenarios you and your training partners can act out. In each exercise, your partner should show clear signs of aggression and a willingness to use violence. Though you know he is your friend, it can still cause an anxious response in your body and mind when he screams and yells in your face that he is going to rip off your head. As he woofs at you, pay attention to not only *what* he is doing but also *how you feel* about it.

Say you feel anxiety surge through your body and those annoying butterflies in your stomach. What do you now? You hit him. Before you start feeling too weak or get too hesitant, step forward and hit or shove him back, hard. This simple response in your training conditions you to recognize the exact moment that you begin feeling overcome with fear and stress. It teaches internal timing, learning to recognize what it feels like when you start to lose control. Then, before it's too late, it teaches you to do something about it. A bully woofs you to verbally assault you into submission. This drill forces you to recognize within yourself when it's time to act, before anxiety, fear and stress turns you to mush or freezes your muscles.

Of course you must be legally justified to strike. If he says, "I'm going to rip your face off," then steps into your space and cocks back his arm, you can legally hit in most jurisdictions. As stated before, be familiar with the laws where you live.

The classics are a true treasure chest of information. But as with all treasures, they are protected well, hidden. It takes effort to get to them, an effort of reading and re-reading, and applying their wisdom to your training. Only then will you see their many layers of knowledge and be able to use them to defend yourself. We have introduced only a few key points from three sources; know that there is much more in them. We encourage you to be a warrior scholar and search them out for yourself.

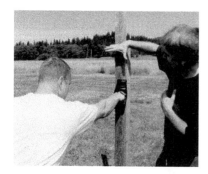

CHAPTER SEVEN

DRILLS

There are many nonthreatening drills in existence that allow fighters to go on autopilot as they do them. This isn't one of them.

The timing drills in this chapter and those discussed and illustrated throughout this book are some of our favorites because they get fast results. Some improve your reaction time, many increase your perception and physical speed, and still others improve your eye/hand coordination. Experiment with all of them, as each one improves your timing in some fashion. While there are other ways to do them, it's advisable to begin by practicing them as described here, and then later add elements from your knowledge and experience.

Since many drills require great speed and power, it's critical to begin with a good warm-up and stretching session. Your body needs to be ready for this kind of training to prevent injury and to achieve optimum results. Let's get going:

Dodge the stick

There are many nonthreatening drills in existence that allow fighters to go on autopilot as they do them. This isn't one of them.

Face a partner who is holding a long stick or a Japanese bo, and stand just inside its reach. Once you are close enough to get hit, you can't move out of range. Your goal is to avoid being hit by moving away from the angle of his attack, but within range. If you moved your body, but your leg got nicked because it trailed behind, take that as a clue that you need to move faster. While this sounds easy, we have a few ways to make it progressively more complicated and challenging.

First, your partner attacks with only two techniques: A horizontal sweep at your head, which you duck under, and a horizontal sweep at your ankles, which you jump over. It's his choice to strike right to left or left to right, and he can break up the rhythm however he wants. He might attack high three times, low once, then high twice, or any other variation. His job is to keep you on your toes. It's also important that he makes a complete pass without hesitation because you want a mind-set of knowing you will get whacked if you don't move out of the way. Start out slowly, and increase the speed only when you are comfortable with the drill. Your objective is to improve until you can avoid nonstop attacks.

Once your chest starts swelling with pride at how good you are, your partner adds a downward, vertical strike, which you sidestep left or right. Once you get comfy with those, he adds diagonal strikes. Expect to eat the occasional blow at this stage (actually, you don't eat it, but you do get whacked in the temple), which is okay because it adds intensity and an accelerated heart rate to the drill.

Practice for 60 seconds and then switch places with your partner.

How you benefit: This drill has four timing benefits: It improves your reaction time when having to move your entire body to avoid a blow; it helps you recognize angles of attack; you learn to stay focused since a poorly timed evasion means you get a painful blow; and you learn to function under stress.

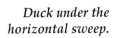
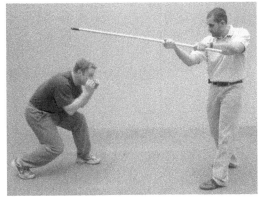

Duck under the horizontal sweep.

Ball dodging

In the movie *Battle Creek Brawl*, Jackie Chan's master tells Jackie to stand with his back to a wall and dodge a bucketful of tennis balls thrown at him. That is what you are going to do here, minus all the diving through the air and summersaults on the floor that Jackie does. It's in your best interest to keep your evasions efficient and realistic. The only equipment needed are a hockey mask or safety goggles, a wall, and a dozen or more tennis balls. Oh, and a training partner with an evil streak.

Stand three or four feet away from a wall that serves as backstop and experiment a little to find a workable distance between you and your partner. While you don't want him to hit you every time, you don't want to make it too easy, either. Try to move only the body part that needs to be "saved" (there shouldn't be enough time to move your entire body, anyway), and strive to remain in balance as you bob, weave and sway. To increase the difficulty, your partner simply steps closer, or you can add a second partner to throw balls at you. If it helps, imagine you are dodging bullets like Neo in the movie *The Matrix*.

Practice dodging a dozen or so balls, and then swap roles with your partner.

How you benefit: Your primary objective is to increase your reaction and timing speed in response to an opponent's offense. But as opposed to the first drill where you moved your entire body, here you move only a specific part, the target, away from your opponent's blow, leaving the rest of your body poised for your response.

Ball slapping

This is similar to Jackie Chan's "Ball dodging," except that you slap the incoming balls out of the way, rather than dodge them. These are fast swats, like you were smacking away a mosquito, except this "mosquito" is about five inches in diameter.

At first, don't dodge, but simply stand in place and swat the balls away from you.

Once you are comfortable with the first phase, swat and dodge at the same time. In the last stage, dodge, swat, and immediately counter with a single technique or combination of your choice in the air. Don't straighten up and then counter, but seize the moment and fire off a return punch or kick no matter how awkward your body position.

Practice dodging a dozen balls and then change places with your training partner.

How you benefit: You learn how to judge distance and timing. Think of the incoming tennis balls as fists screaming toward your face or body that you must intercept not a second too soon or a second too late. You will discover that full-power blocks, especially the traditional types where one arm crosses in front of the other, are just too slow against a fast pitch. It's much faster to simply move the force aside or evade it.

Back to the wall

Stand with your back three or four inches away from a wall, facing your training partner who stands just outside of punching range. On his whim, he steps in and attacks with single hand techniques that you block or deflect. For now, don't counter but just observe the attack and defend accordingly. You can't use footwork, but you can use your hands and arms, and you can shift your weight to the sides, duck, or lean in any direction.

When this gets easy for you, your partner steps closer, just inside punching range. This forces you to concentrate harder and move even faster, responding the same as before. Continue working on this stage until it feels comfortable.

Return to the first stage, but this time, block, and then counter immediately with a fast hand technique. When you get comfy with this, your partner steps in closer again and launches his attacks from inside punching range.

Practice 2 to 3, 1-minute rounds of each stage.

How you benefit: This drill helps you perceive early warning signs of different attacks. You see your attacker's eyes, shoulders, elbows, and waist without focusing on any specific one. Don't second-guess, but maintain an empty mind (Mushin) and defend instinctively. Because you can't step away from the close attacker, your reaction time becomes a critical issue. When you get hit because you erred, ask your partner to repeat the same attack a few times so you can find a better response. Always correct your errors, so you ingrain the best response into your subconscious.

Touch and go

Full-contact sport fighters as well as street brawlers often hold their arms tight in front of them as a way to defend against in-coming blows. While it's a good idea to cover up, doing so can make it difficult to *see* what is going on, though you can certainly *feel* all the hitting. Here is a timing drill that helps you get out of this situation when you feel the moment is right. Begin by gearing up with boxing gloves, shin pads and headgear.

Get close to your training buddy, cover your head with your guard and prepare to get hit. At first, your partner only fires left and right hooks, one every five seconds. Your objective is to time your counter to hit back an instant after you get hit. For example, the moment you feel a blow to the left side of your guard, return a fast left hook of your own while maintaining tight cover. Your partner waits five seconds and then attacks with a hook to the right side of your head, which hits your guard. You immediately counter with a right hook to his head. Though you might occasionally hit your partner's punching arm, with a little practice your counter punch will land neatly in his surprised face. To keep things simple, he should not counter your counter, as the drill will just turn into a brawl. One person feeds the hooks, the other counters. As your skill improves, your partner can include hooks to your body, too.

When you are ready for the final stage, your partner unleashes a combination of punches on your closed guard, and your task is to time a counter wherever possible.

Practice 3 to 4, 2-minute rounds, alternating roles with your partner each round.

How you benefit: This drill teaches you to take advantage of a small but distinct window of opportunity to help you get out of a tough jam by hitting your attacker on the same side he just hit you. Since your fists are covering your head and eyes, you train to react to the *feeling* of where you just got hit. If your timing is right on the mark, he will be open because he is thinking about where to hit you next, as most fighters tend to alternate arms when doing combinations.

Surprise attack

For this drill, which we adapted from kali instructor Mike Inay, you need at least five people: three attackers, one defender and one coordinator. Here is how you set it up.

Three attackers stand side-by-side and face a defender positioned just one step away from them. The fourth person, the coordinator, stands behind the defender. His job is to tell the attackers what to do by using hand signals or by silently demonstrating the technique. Since the defender is looking the other way, he doesn't know which attacker is being signaled or what technique is being ordered. Therefore, he must stay alert and ready to react with speed.

You can make this drill as complex or as simple as you like. Here are a few pointers for maximum effect:

- Each attacker is numbered from left to right to make it easy for the coordinator who holds up one to three fingers to indicate who he wants to attack.

- Though it's sometimes confusing at first, you can number the attacks too: 1 is a jab, 2 is a reverse punch, 3 is a roundhouse kick, and so on.

- Some coordinators like to pantomime or demonstrate the technique. He should pantomime just enough of the technique so the attacker understands what he is to do. For example, he lifts his rear leg in a partial front kick. If he does too much of the move, the defender can guess the technique from the sound.

- Another option is to indicate the target to be struck. The coordinator touches his knee to indicate a low sidekick, or touches his stomach to indicate a reverse punch.

- The coordinator can clinch his fist to indicate a "Go!" sign.

Practice 10-15 attacks and then switch roles. The drill concludes when all five fighters have defended.

How you benefit: This is a stressful drill with multiple attackers, unknown attacks, and a pace that is controlled by the coordinator. But stress is good. After only a few sessions, your reaction time and defense will improve tremendously.

Karate-ball

This is one of co-author Demeere's favorites. Carry a volleyball ball onto a racquetball court (after explaining to the staff about the weird thing you are about to do so they don't call the police) and prepare to play a game of racquetball using punches, backfists, knees, elbows, and kicks instead of a racquet. No flailing is allowed, only hard hitting with good form. You have to run, jump, twist and turn each time to hit the bouncing ball correctly and at the right moment.

Go for as many 2- to 3-minute rounds as you can without becoming sloppy with fatigue. Rest for a minute between each round.

How you benefit: There is a tremendous amount of timing and distancing involved as you continuously determine where the ball is heading and which technique best fits the moment. The benefits of this drill also overlap to multiple opponent training. You must perceive, analyze and then adapt your techniques to windows of opportunity as they present themselves from a variety of angles and directions. The speed of the bouncing ball increases the difficulty while quickly improving your timing and footwork.

Stop the bag

To warm-up for this drill, do three or four two-minute rounds of only linear techniques -- straight punches and straight kicks -- on a heavy bag. Once you have a little sweat happening and you have established good rhythm, give the bag a hard front kick to get it swinging. Let the first swing pass by but when it swings towards you again, stop its forward momentum with a front kick, reverse punch, jab, sidekick or any other linear technique. Try to hit it when it's almost perpendicular to the floor, and brace yourself for a good impact.

The next step is to use circular techniques: hooking punches, roundhouse kicks, crescent kicks and so on. Practice a few reps in the air of each technique you intend to use and then commence doing them on the bag after you get it swinging sideways. For example, as the bag swings toward your right, fire a right roundhouse kick into it, stopping the bag dead in its tracks. You might find that this is harder to do with your hand techniques than with your kicks, but keep training and soon the power will be yours.

When you get proficient with circular blows against a swinging bag, try free sparring it using your favorite single techniques and combinations to stop the momentum no matter which way it's moving.

Push the bag away and time your punch to land at the right moment.

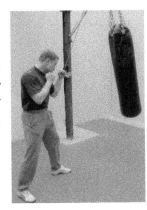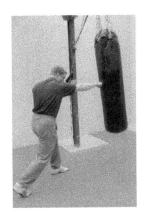

Practice 4 or 5, 2-minute rounds.

Warning: Because of the massive amount of kinetic energy involved, small errors can lead to big injuries. A wrist held at the wrong angle, for example, will sprain or break when hitting full power. Think of it as nature's way of telling you that you screwed up. Start out slowly, swing the bag slightly at first, and train for precise form. Increase the swing as your skill level improves.

How you benefit: The drill trains your ability to hit on a collision course with a moving target, one with mass and weight similar to a human's. It's definitely a different feel than hitting a focus mitt because unless you hit it with good technique, solid power and with a sound foundation, the heavy bag can knock you off balance and disrupt your stance. With this drill, you develop knockout power by learning to time your techniques into an onrushing attacker.

The fan drill

Retired army Lieutenant Colonel Dave Grossman, author of *On Killing, On Combat* and others, told us about a dry firing drill he uses with a handgun. In the event you aren't a gun aficionado, know that "dry firing" means there are no bullets in the weapon when the trigger is pulled. *NO* bullets in the gun. The gun is *empty*. Is the gun loaded? Absolutely not. We hope that is clear.

The "shooter" attaches two, one-inch pieces of tape to one blade of a large, wall-mounted fan, a fan that whirls at variable speeds. One piece of tape is applied at the blade's halfway point and another at its tip. The shooter, armed with an *empty* gun, points his weapon at the spinning blades. He doesn't follow the spinning tape while making circles with the barrel of the gun, but rather focuses at 12 o'clock and "fires" when the tape crosses that point. The tape at the half point on the blade is easier to shoot since it's moving seemingly more slowly than the one at the tip. Colonel Grossman says that at first it seems virtually impossible, but with continuous practice one can quickly improve timing so that he can "shoot" the tape each time it passes.

This is a wonderful timing drill that can be adapted easily to the martial arts by simply using striking techniques instead of dry firing an empty gun. Each time the tape passes 12 o'clock, jab it, backfist it, or flick it with your fingers as if poking an eye. You can even reverse punch it if you have the speed. To be clear, you are striking *at* the tape from at least 12 inches away, not actually hitting it, unless you want to be called Lefty for the rest of your life (or Righty, depending on which hand turns into red wall splatter). If you possess killer-fast kicks, give them try, too. But move back farther.

Start out hitting at the tape attached at the halfway point, and after you can do that easily, advance to striking at the one attached to the blade's tip. If you get too systematic with your strikes, that is, you hit each time the tape passes, you become a pumping piston and there is no timing benefit to the drill. Begin by striking at every fifth pass, then fourth, and then third. About the time you get comfortable – you can hit it easily every third pass – you are then ready for random hitting. Using the same stance, look away for a second or two, and then look back at the fan, striking at the tape the next time it points to 12 o'clock.

Once you can do it at low speed, advance to medium. If you have a ceiling fan that has variable speeds, lie on your back under it and attack using as many techniques as you can from that position.

Practice with each hand in sets of 10 reps.

How you benefit: This is an especially dynamic drill that develops your ability to hit a target (think of the passing blade as an opening) and do so with great speed. It works your visual recognition, reaction time and muscle speed. Begin the exercise using your lead arm and lead foot techniques, since they are closer to the target and therefore faster. When you are ready, use your rear hand and back leg.

Pin the glove to the wall

Here is another drill from Lt. Col. Dave Grossman, one he learned from a friend who trained with knives. Armed with a knife, the man would stand in his fighting stance and face toward his wife who held a yardstick out to her side. At her discretion, she would drop the stick and he would try to pin the stick to a wall before it dropped to the floor. (We can only assume this was done outside next to a shed or tree, and not in the kitchen). The less distance the stick dropped, as measured in inches, the higher his score.

To modify this for martial arts, get a training partner to hold a glove against a wall about as high as your head. Face the wall and assume your fighting stance, close enough to touch it without moving your feet, and stand alert and ready to react with whatever technique you choose when the glove drops. When the glove is released, snap out your technique to pin it to the wall. Though there is a risk of hitting the hard surface and injuring the hand, we use a wall or post because it helps us to develop control. Other times when we want to hit full force, the glove is held against a standing or hanging bag.

When you feel you are ready, move back a little so you have to stretch forward farther to pin the glove. When you can eventually pin the glove to the wall at a distance where you have to step forward, you have arrived, almost. How do you know when you have arrived all the way?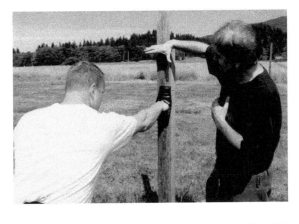
When you can lunge forward and pin a dropped dime to the wall with your index finger. Christensen *claims* he can do this and make change. He *says* he can lunge toward a dropped dime, replace it with a nickel, pin the nickel to the wall, pocket the dime, and hand his training partner a second nickel, all in a split second. Not surprisingly, no one has ever seen him do this.

Practice with each hand in sets of 10 reps.

How you benefit: This drill sharpens your reaction speed to a dropped glove. Think of it as your opponent's hand dropping momentarily, giving you a window of opportunity to punch the resultant opening. Should you react and move to slowly, the glove drops all the way and you hit open air, or the wall should you not stop in time.

Yardstick

Let's stay with the yardstick drill mentioned in the last exercise and look at a fun way to test and improve your reaction speed. You just need a partner and a yardstick. A ruler works, too, but you have to be quick.

Your partner holds the yardstick between his thumb and forefinger at the highest number, 36 inches. To ensure that you don't cheat by following the dropped yardstick with your hand, rest your wrist on a table or the back of a chair. With that same hand, position your thumb on one side of the one-inch mark at the bottom of the yardstick and forefinger on the other side. Your fingers are an inch apart and not touching the stick. Once you are ready, your partner releases the stick without warning and you respond by pinching both fingers together as quickly as possible to stop the stick's fall. Write down the number on the stick (the inches mark) where your fingers catch it. Use the following chart to determine your reaction time in seconds and milliseconds.

Distance of catch	Reaction Time (in seconds)
2 in (~5 cm)	0.10 sec (100 ms)
4 in (~10 cm)	0.14 sec (140 ms)
6 in (~15 cm)	0.17 sec (170 ms)
8 in (~20 cm)	0.20 sec (200 ms)
10 in (~25.5 cm)	0.23 sec (230 ms)
12 in (~30.5 cm)	0.25 sec (250 ms)
17 in (~43 cm)	0.30 sec (300 ms)
24 in (~61 cm)	0.35 sec (350 ms)
31 in (~79 cm)	0.40 sec (400 ms)
39 in (~99 cm)	0.45 sec (450 ms)
48 in (~123 cm)	0.50 sec (500 ms)
69 in (~175 cm)	0.60 sec (600 ms

Your partner should avoid letting go of the stick rhythmically, such as every three seconds. Instead, he should drop it between one and five seconds. Sometimes he drops it at one second, other times after four seconds, and so on. After three to five tries, calculate your average score.

(In case you were wondering, no, you can't do the exercise by yourself, dropping it with one hand and catching it with the other.)

Test yourself when you are rested and fresh.

How you benefit: This drill enhances your ability to perceive and react to a stimulus with speed. Unlike many other drills, you get an immediate feedback as to how you are doing with each repetition.

React to the string

Your partner stands behind a heavy bag or a mannequin bag, reaches around it and twirls a 24- to 30-inch piece of string. Your job is to stand in your fighting stance and punch the bag without getting entangled in the string on the way in or the way out.

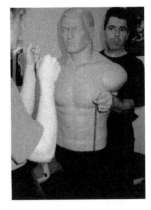

Tip: Watch as the string passes a point of your choice, usually 12 o'clock, and punch out and snap it back quickly. At first, your partner twirls the string as slowly as gravity allows, but then increases the speed once you get the feel for it.

Practice 1 to 2 sets of 10 reps of each technique. Stop when you are fatigued.

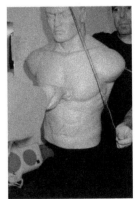

How you benefit: This develops timing, speed and especially your ability to concentrate. Do you have fast kicks? Try them on this drill.

Hand mitts hitting drill

For this classic drill you need a partner and two hand-held punching mitts. Your partner moves around, slowly at first, holding the pads down at his sides or behind him. When he suddenly presents one to you in striking range, you attack with the best technique given its position. Your partner should present the mitts in different positions -- palm side up, down, and to the side -- to get you to use different techniques. If you are in kicking range, kick it; if you are closer, use a hand technique. He also varies the levels from low to high. Sometimes he allows you to come close and other times he forces you to use footwork to close the gap. A good partner pays close attention to you and pushes you to stay focused. If you drop your guard or don't cover up properly when attacking, he slaps you with the mitts. To make the drill even more fun, try these variations:

- Your partner holds up two mitts to get you to make a combination.

- Turn down the lights to make the mitts harder to see

- Close your eyes and follow your partner by listening to the sound of his footwork. He picks a random moment to shout, "Go!" signaling you to open your eyes and react to the mitt(s) he presents.

- As soon as your partner sees you launch your attack, he steps back to force you to go after it. He doesn't jerk the mitt away when he steps, but keeps it at the same position, though it moves back with him.

Practice for 2 to 3, 2-minute rounds, changing roles after every round.

How you benefit: This drill helps you to quickly perceive a target opportunity, decide which technique best fits the moment, and then move as quick as a blink.

Rhythm kicking drill

Here is a simple drill that works for both beginners and advanced fighters. Square off with your partner and launch a roundhouse kick at him. He blocks it and then counters with a roundhouse of his own as you retract your kicking leg. Don't block his counter. Then it's his turn to throw a roundhouse kick, which you block and counter with a roundhouse of your own. He doesn't block your counter. Continue back and forth for 10 reps each.

Practice 2 set of 10 reps each kick on both sides.

How you benefit: The concept is to train yourself to counter as your partner *retracts* his attack, a timing moment when he is at his weakest. Though the roundhouse kick is mentioned here, you can use any technique you want, including punches. Just be sure to counter on the retraction. You also benefit by getting in lots of reps with whichever technique you choose to use.

Timing a feint

Start sparring with your partner, using whatever rules and techniques you decide upon. As you move about, throw a couple of jabs at an even pace, say three seconds apart, each at the same speed. Then feint a third one, freeze it at the end of the fake for a quarter second, then complete the movement by whacking him in the face. The short pause in your rhythm disrupts your opponent's mental balance and clears a path for that third, completed jab. Having been conditioned, he reacts to the feint by blocking or dodging, which is exactly what you want him to do so that he is open to your real jab.

Though this works exceptionally well with the jab, you can use your sparring session to try other punches and your kicks to see if you can consistently trick your partner into falling for the feint. Focus on one technique per round or include several.

Practice 3 to 4, 2-minute rounds.

How you benefit: Establishing a rhythm and then breaking it is a classic way to apply offensive timing. It's actually more difficult to do than it might seem, so plan to spend time getting it polished. Knowing when to change the rhythm of a set-up teaches you to seize a window of opportunity that you force open.

Baiting

In the previous drill, you wanted him to think that you were going to execute the same technique you had just delivered two or three times. With "Baiting," you want him to believe you are done hitting him with a barrage of techniques, but you aren't. You have one more for him.

Begin by sparring. Say you throw a jab-jab-cross combination. Just as you finish the cross, hesitate for a second so he thinks you are through with your blitz. Then fire a powerful hook into his face. To make it appear even more like you are finished punching, shift your weight back a little after your cross punch. The key is to make him believe you have finished your combination so that he lowers his guard a little or tries to counter. At that instant, plow your hook punch into him.

Most often when your opponent uses a combination, his techniques machinegun you for a second or two, then it's over as he moves away. Many fighters are accustomed to this rhythm or pattern, and automatically relax or attempt to counter when their opponent stops. Great. That is what you want your opponent to think. By making him believe that you are finished and about to move away, you have created a moment, a pause, in his mind, one in which he is vulnerable to that hook. This works so well that even in training when you both know that the goal is to bait each other, you still fall for it. Once you have a feel for the jab, jab, cross, pause, and then hook punch, devise your own attack, using your preferred techniques to attack, pause and then hit.

Practice 3 to 4, 2-minute rounds with one or several combinations.

How you benefit: By working with the concept of baiting, you learn to create timing opportunities by manipulating your opponent's mind.

Catch the rabbit

In this sparring drill, you often feel as if you were trying to catch a rabbit, as your opponent jumps about and zigzags out of the way every time you think you got him. Sometimes you get so frustrated that if you could catch the "rabbit" you would happily skin him and throw him on a barbeque. Though skinning and cooking aren't advised, try your best in this drill to catch your evasive partner.

As you spar, your partner's job is to attack by scooting quickly in and out of range, focusing more on speed than power as he tags you with punches and kicks without him getting hit. Against such a fighter, it's hard for you to score a one-punch knockout because he is scurrying about like a bunny. He moves so quickly and hits you from so many different angles, continuously forcing you into a new OODA loop, that you don't have time or opportunity to establish a solid base and hit him with a power shot.

So don't try. Instead of counting on that one, devastating technique, work on either pre-empting, by hitting him as he advances on you, or by following him as he tries to run away. Use quick kicks and jabs, techniques that are less powerful but serve to open the door for an opportunity to slam in harder ones.

Practice 2 to 3, 2-minute rounds, reversing roles every time.

How you benefit: This drill benefits you in three ways: It reduces your reaction time to specific attacks; it improves your timing by forcing you to instantly choose which of the three typical reference points to use (before, during or after the attack. See Chapter One); and it helps you with tactical timing (which weapon best suits the moment of opportunity)

When it's your turn to play the rabbit, you learn to time your initial move to close the gap without getting hit. You also learn how many fast attacks you can deliver before it's time to get out of there. Should you stay in front of your partner too long, you get clobbered. Should you move away too soon, you miss precious opportunities to hit.

Conclusion

A fight, whether in the street, a training facility, or in a ring, consists of timing moments. It begins with the best moment to throw the first blow and it ends with the best moment to throw the last. When timing is optimum in a street fight or full-contact competition, the fist blow and the last blow are the same blow. But when it lasts longer, a fight can consist of a dozen, even a hundred or more timing moments. To use current vernacular: It's all about timing.

Timing is involved even when training alone: executing reps in the air, on the heavy bags, and working on your forms. When practicing a kick and punch combination in the air, you must decide when to launch the punch after the kick. When working on a heavy swinging bag, you need to hit it at the precise moment to maximize your impact and minimize spraining a joint. When practicing a form, you need to consider when and how long to pause, when to turn and when to attack that imaginary foe sneaking up behind you.

But never is timing more important than when facing a live opponent, in practice, in competition and on the street.

So many martial artists practice only to develop the three elements of speed, power and precise body mechanics. All good. All critical. But timing is the fourth critical element, the too often neglected one. In fact, as we have discussed throughout this book and as we have quoted from many great fighters and instructors, timing is arguably the most important. Yes, it's good to be fast; yes, it's good to be powerful; and yes, precise body mechanics are mandatory. But if you can't find the right moment, if you can't seize the window of opportunity, if you can't find the hole in your opponent's defenses to get that fast, strong and well-formed technique to the target, all is lost.

We hope that this book has given you, no matter what your style, some food for thought in your training, some valuable concepts to mull about, and many beneficial drills, all to improve your ability to slam your offense or defense into that bullseye at precisely the right moment.

Index

A

adrenaline 24
adrenal stress 24
age 25, 140–141
amygdala 20
angle 99–100
angles 77
arousal 24
auditory stimulus 34
A Book of Five Rings 268–272

B

baiting 130, 288
balance 205–209
bear hug 67
biomechanical structure 110
blocks 40
body manipulation 68
body punches 238–241
body targets 239
boxer's stance 110
boxing 110
Boyd, Colonel John 26
Boyd's Cycle 27, 77
brain 19, 22
breakfall 171

C

car 195
centerline 104–112
central nervous system 19
checklist 176–177
circles of influence 83
clinch 97
close-range weapons 84
close range 83
closing the gap 246–251
cognitive load 25
combinations 36, 138
competition 36
concentration 59

D

deescalation stance 90
defensive response 184
deflecting 169–170
distance 88, 99
distraction 248–249
double tap 137–138
drawing 70, 150, 234–235
drills 39
duck 41
dynamic tension training 142

E

elbow and knee range 95
environmental obstacles 164
environmental weapon 193
escape 64, 175
evading 168, 170
expectation 24
experience 157

F

faking 70
falling 171
fast-twitch muscle fibers 21
fatigue 25
feinting 70, 127–128, 287
fighting ranges 82, 82–92
floating ribs 240
flow 59–61
focus 64
footwork 34, 63, 102–104, 162
force 191
framing 102

G

gender 141
grappling 104, 205
grappling range 83, 95–98
group attacks 217–222
guard 114
gun 209–212

H

hand mitts 286
Heal, Captain Sid 27
Hick's Law 46–47
high kick 242–243

I

indicator 184–185
initiative 36
injuries 140–141
insert 179
instinctive reactions 37

K

kicking range 92
knife defense 212–214

L

law enforcement 48
levels 129
limb positioning 119
lines of attack 76–77
liver 239
long range 83

M

medium range 83
military 48
mirror 155
monitoring 184
multiple opponents 214
muscle fibers 21
muscular tension 24
mushin 53–57

N

natural blocks 40
nervous system 22
no-mind 53–57

O

obstacles 64
offensive response 185
OODA loop 26–29, 44, 78, 101, 122,
        131, 215, 255–256
overreach 96

P

parrying 169
perception 23
phases of timing 71–73
planned group attacks 217
point of unbalance 97
positioning 98
posture 112
power 149, 152
pre-emptive strike 167
programming 23
punching range 93–94

R

ranges 83–92
range diagram 83
reach 88–89
reaction time 23–24, 132
realism 32
reflexes 37
response option 47
response selection 23
response time 23–24
reverse punch 89
rhythm 287
roundhouse angle kick 232

S

scenario training 31, 33, 164
self-defense 31, 48, 181
sensation 23
senses 19
set-up 35, 137
side stance 114
slap kick 91
slow-twitch muscle fibers 21

solar plexus 239
speed 21, 134–139, 142, 154
spine 107
stance 63, 102, 110–117, 249
stimulus 22–25
stress 20

T

Tai Chi Chuan Classics 260
target 21
telegraphing 22
The Art of War 264
threatening 181–187
trained responses 39–40
training log 147–148
trapping 131–133

U

unplanned group attacks 221

V

verbal tactics 69

W

warning 26
weapons 64, 188–191, 216
weight distribution 116
weight training 142, 149

NOTES

NOTES

NOTES

NOTES

NOTES

ABOUT THE AUTHORS

Loren W. Christensen began studying the martial arts in 1965. Over the years he has earned 10 black belts, seven in karate, two in jujitsu and one in arnis. He used his training as a military policeman in Saigon, Vietnam, a police officer for 25 years in Portland, Oregon, and as a karate tournament competitor, capturing 53 wins.

As a free-lance writer, Loren has authored 27 books (half of them on the martial arts) including *On Combat: The Psychology and Physiology of Deadly Conflict in War and in Peace* and *Warriors: On Living with Courage, Discipline and Honor*, dozens of magazine articles, and edited a newspaper for nearly eight years. He has recently starred in five instructional martial arts videos. Retired from police work, Loren now writes full time, teaches martial arts to a small group of students, and gives seminars on the martial arts, police defensive tactics, and verbal judo.

To contact Loren, visit his website LWC Books at www.lwcbooks.com.

§

Wim Demeere began training at the age of 14, studying the grappling arts of judo and jujitsu for several years before turning to the kick/punch arts of traditional kung fu and full-contact fighting. Over the years he has studied a broad range of other fighting styles, including muay Thai, kali, pentjak silat and shootfighting. Since the late 1990s, he has been studying tai chi chuan and its martial applications.

Wim's competitive years saw him win four national titles and a bronze medal at the 1995 World Wushu Championships. In 2001, he became the national coach of the Belgian Wushu fighting team.

A full-time personal trainer in his native country of Belgium, Wim instructs both business executives and athletes in nutrition, strength and endurance, and a variety of martial arts styles. He has managed a corporate wellness center and regularly gives lectures and workshops in the corporate world.

You can contact Wim through his website The Grinding Shop at www.grindingshop.com

Loren and Wim co-authored *The Fighter's Body: An Owner's Manual: Your Guide to Diet, Nutrition, Exercise and Excellence in the Martial Arts*

BOOKS FROM YMAA

6 HEALING MOVEMENTS
101 REFLECTIONS ON TAI CHI CHUAN
108 INSIGHTS INTO TAI CHI CHUAN
ADVANCING IN TAE KWON DO
ANALYSIS OF SHAOLIN CHIN NA 2ND ED
ANCIENT CHINESE WEAPONS
ART OF HOJO UNDO
ARTHRITIS RELIEF, 3RD ED.
BACK PAIN RELIEF, 2ND ED.
BAGUAZHANG, 2ND ED.
CARDIO KICKBOXING ELITE
CHIN NA IN GROUND FIGHTING
CHINESE FAST WRESTLING
CHINESE FITNESS
CHINESE TUI NA MASSAGE
CHOJUN
COMPREHENSIVE APPLICATIONS OF SHAOLIN
    CHIN NA
CONFLICT COMMUNICATION
CROCODILE AND THE CRANE: A NOVEL
CUTTING SEASON: A XENON PEARL MARTIAL ARTS
    THRILLER
DEFENSIVE TACTICS
DESHI: A CONNOR BURKE MARTIAL ARTS THRILLER
DIRTY GROUND
DR. WU'S HEAD MASSAGE
DUKKHA HUNGRY GHOSTS
DUKKHA REVERB
DUKKHA, THE SUFFERING: AN EYE FOR AN EYE
DUKKHA UNLOADED
ENZAN: THE FAR MOUNTAIN, A CONNOR BURKE MARTIAL
    ARTS THRILLER
ESSENCE OF SHAOLIN WHITE CRANE
EXPLORING TAI CHI
FACING VIOLENCE
FIGHT BACK
FIGHT LIKE A PHYSICIST
THE FIGHTER'S BODY
FIGHTER'S FACT BOOK
FIGHTER'S FACT BOOK 2
FIGHTING THE PAIN RESISTANT ATTACKER
FIRST DEFENSE
FORCE DECISIONS: A CITIZENS GUIDE
FOX BORROWS THE TIGER'S AWE
INSIDE TAI CHI
KAGE: THE SHADOW, A CONNOR BURKE MARTIAL ARTS
    THRILLER
KATA AND THE TRANSMISSION OF KNOWLEDGE
KRAV MAGA PROFESSIONAL TACTICS
KRAV MAGA WEAPON DEFENSES
LITTLE BLACK BOOK OF VIOLENCE
LIUHEBAFA FIVE CHARACTER SECRETS
MARTIAL ARTS ATHLETE
MARTIAL ARTS INSTRUCTION
MARTIAL WAY AND ITS VIRTUES
MASK OF THE KING
MEDITATIONS ON VIOLENCE
MIND/BODY FITNESS
THE MIND INSIDE TAI CHI
THE MIND INSIDE YANG STYLE TAI CHI CHUAN
MUGAI RYU
NATURAL HEALING WITH QIGONG
NORTHERN SHAOLIN SWORD, 2ND ED.
OKINAWA'S COMPLETE KARATE SYSTEM: ISSHIN RYU
POWER BODY
PRINCIPLES OF TRADITIONAL CHINESE MEDICINE
QIGONG FOR HEALTH & MARTIAL ARTS 2ND ED.

QIGONG FOR LIVING
QIGONG FOR TREATING COMMON AILMENTS
QIGONG MASSAGE
QIGONG MEDITATION: EMBRYONIC BREATHING
QIGONG MEDITATION: SMALL CIRCULATION
QIGONG, THE SECRET OF YOUTH: DA MO'S CLASSICS
QUIET TEACHER: A XENON PEARL MARTIAL ARTS THRILLER
RAVEN'S WARRIOR
REDEMPTION
ROOT OF CHINESE QIGONG, 2ND ED.
SCALING FORCE
SENSEI: A CONNOR BURKE MARTIAL ARTS THRILLER
SHIHAN TE: THE BUNKAI OF KATA
SHIN GI TAI: KARATE TRAINING FOR BODY, MIND, AND
    SPIRIT
SIMPLE CHINESE MEDICINE
SIMPLE QIGONG EXERCISES FOR HEALTH, 3RD ED.
SIMPLIFIED TAI CHI CHUAN, 2ND ED.
SIMPLIFIED TAI CHI FOR BEGINNERS
SOLO TRAINING
SOLO TRAINING 2
SUDDEN DAWN: THE EPIC JOURNEY OF BODHIDHARMA
SUNRISE TAI CHI
SUNSET TAI CHI
SURVIVING ARMED ASSAULTS
TAE KWON DO: THE KOREAN MARTIAL ART
TAEKWONDO BLACK BELT POOMSAE
TAEKWONDO: A PATH TO EXCELLENCE
TAEKWONDO: ANCIENT WISDOM FOR THE MODERN
    WARRIOR
TAEKWONDO: DEFENSES AGAINST WEAPONS
TAEKWONDO: SPIRIT AND PRACTICE
TAO OF BIOENERGETICS
TAI CHI BALL QIGONG: FOR HEALTH AND MARTIAL ARTS
TAI CHI BALL WORKOUT FOR BEGINNERS
TAI CHI BOOK
TAI CHI CHIN NA: THE SEIZING ART OF TAI CHI CHUAN,
    2ND ED.
TAI CHI CHUAN CLASSICAL YANG STYLE, 2ND ED.
TAI CHI CHUAN MARTIAL APPLICATIONS
TAI CHI CHUAN MARTIAL POWER, 3RD ED.
TAI CHI CONNECTIONS
TAI CHI DYNAMICS
TAI CHI QIGONG, 3RD ED.
TAI CHI SECRETS OF THE ANCIENT MASTERS
TAI CHI SECRETS OF THE WU & LI STYLES
TAI CHI SECRETS OF THE WU STYLE
TAI CHI SECRETS OF THE YANG STYLE
TAI CHI SWORD: CLASSICAL YANG STYLE, 2ND ED.
TAI CHI SWORD FOR BEGINNERS
TAI CHI WALKING
TAIJIQUAN THEORY OF DR. YANG, JWING-MING
TENGU: THE MOUNTAIN GOBLIN, A CONNOR BURKE MAR-
    TIAL ARTS THRILLER
TIMING IN THE FIGHTING ARTS
TRADITIONAL CHINESE HEALTH SECRETS
TRADITIONAL TAEKWONDO
TRAINING FOR SUDDEN VIOLENCE
WAY OF KATA
WAY OF KENDO AND KENJITSU
WAY OF SANCHIN KATA
WAY TO BLACK BELT
WESTERN HERBS FOR MARTIAL ARTISTS
WILD GOOSE QIGONG
WOMAN'S QIGONG GUIDE
XINGYIQUAN

DVDS FROM YMAA

ADVANCED PRACTICAL CHIN NA IN-DEPTH

ANALYSIS OF SHAOLIN CHIN NA

ATTACK THE ATTACK

BAGUAZHANG: EMEI BAGUAZHANG

CHEN STYLE TAIJIQUAN

CHIN NA IN-DEPTH COURSES 1—4

CHIN NA IN-DEPTH COURSES 5—8

CHIN NA IN-DEPTH COURSES 9—12

FACING VIOLENCE: 7 THINGS A MARTIAL ARTIST MUST KNOW

FIVE ANIMAL SPORTS

JOINT LOCKS

KNIFE DEFENSE: TRADITIONAL TECHNIQUES AGAINST A DAGGER

KUNG FU BODY CONDITIONING 1

KUNG FU BODY CONDITIONING 2

KUNG FU FOR KIDS

KUNG FU FOR TEENS

INFIGHTING

LOGIC OF VIOLENCE

MERIDIAN QIGONG

NEIGONG FOR MARTIAL ARTS

NORTHERN SHAOLIN SWORD : SAN CAI JIAN, KUN WU JIAN, QI MEN JIAN

QIGONG MASSAGE

QIGONG FOR HEALING

QIGONG FOR LONGEVITY

QIGONG FOR WOMEN

SABER FUNDAMENTAL TRAINING

SAI TRAINING AND SEQUENCES

SANCHIN KATA: TRADITIONAL TRAINING FOR KARATE POWER

SHAOLIN KUNG FU FUNDAMENTAL TRAINING: COURSES 1 & 2

SHAOLIN LONG FIST KUNG FU: BASIC SEQUENCES

SHAOLIN LONG FIST KUNG FU: INTERMEDIATE SEQUENCES

SHAOLIN LONG FIST KUNG FU: ADVANCED SEQUENCES 1

SHAOLIN LONG FIST KUNG FU: ADVANCED SEQUENCES 2

SHAOLIN SABER: BASIC SEQUENCES

SHAOLIN STAFF: BASIC SEQUENCES

SHAOLIN WHITE CRANE GONG FU BASIC TRAINING: COURSES 1 & 2

SHAOLIN WHITE CRANE GONG FU BASIC TRAINING: COURSES 3 & 4

SHUAI JIAO: KUNG FU WRESTLING

SIMPLE QIGONG EXERCISES FOR ARTHRITIS RELIEF

SIMPLE QIGONG EXERCISES FOR BACK PAIN RELIEF

SIMPLIFIED TAI CHI CHUAN: 24 & 48 POSTURES

SIMPLIFIED TAI CHI FOR BEGINNERS 48

SUNRISE TAI CHI

SUNSET TAI CHI

SWORD: FUNDAMENTAL TRAINING

TAEKWONDO KORYO POOMSAE

TAI CHI BALL QIGONG: COURSES 1 & 2

TAI CHI BALL QIGONG: COURSES 3 & 4

TAI CHI BALL WORKOUT FOR BEGINNERS

TAI CHI CHUAN CLASSICAL YANG STYLE

TAI CHI CONNECTIONS

TAI CHI ENERGY PATTERNS

TAI CHI FIGHTING SET

TAI CHI PUSHING HANDS: COURSES 1 & 2

TAI CHI PUSHING HANDS: COURSES 3 & 4

TAI CHI SWORD: CLASSICAL YANG STYLE

TAI CHI SWORD FOR BEGINNERS

TAI CHI SYMBOL: YIN YANG STICKING HANDS

TAIJI & SHAOLIN STAFF: FUNDAMENTAL TRAINING

TAIJI CHIN NA IN-DEPTH

TAIJI 37 POSTURES MARTIAL APPLICATIONS

TAIJI SABER CLASSICAL YANG STYLE

TAIJI WRESTLING

TRAINING FOR SUDDEN VIOLENCE

UNDERSTANDING QIGONG 1: WHAT IS QI? • HUMAN QI CIRCULATORY SYSTEM

UNDERSTANDING QIGONG 2: KEY POINTS • QIGONG BREATHING

UNDERSTANDING QIGONG 3: EMBRYONIC BREATHING

UNDERSTANDING QIGONG 4: FOUR SEASONS QIGONG

UNDERSTANDING QIGONG 5: SMALL CIRCULATION

UNDERSTANDING QIGONG 6: MARTIAL QIGONG BREATHING

WHITE CRANE HARD & SOFT QIGONG

WUDANG KUNG FU: FUNDAMENTAL TRAINING

WUDANG SWORD

WUDANG TAIJIQUAN

XINGYIQUAN

YANG TAI CHI FOR BEGINNERS

YMAA 25 YEAR ANNIVERSARY DVD

more products available from . . .

YMAA Publication Center, Inc. 楊氏東方文化出版中心

1-800-669-8892 • info@ymaa.com • www.ymaa.com